an introduction to
AROMATHERAPY

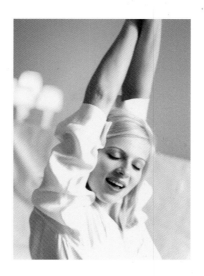

p

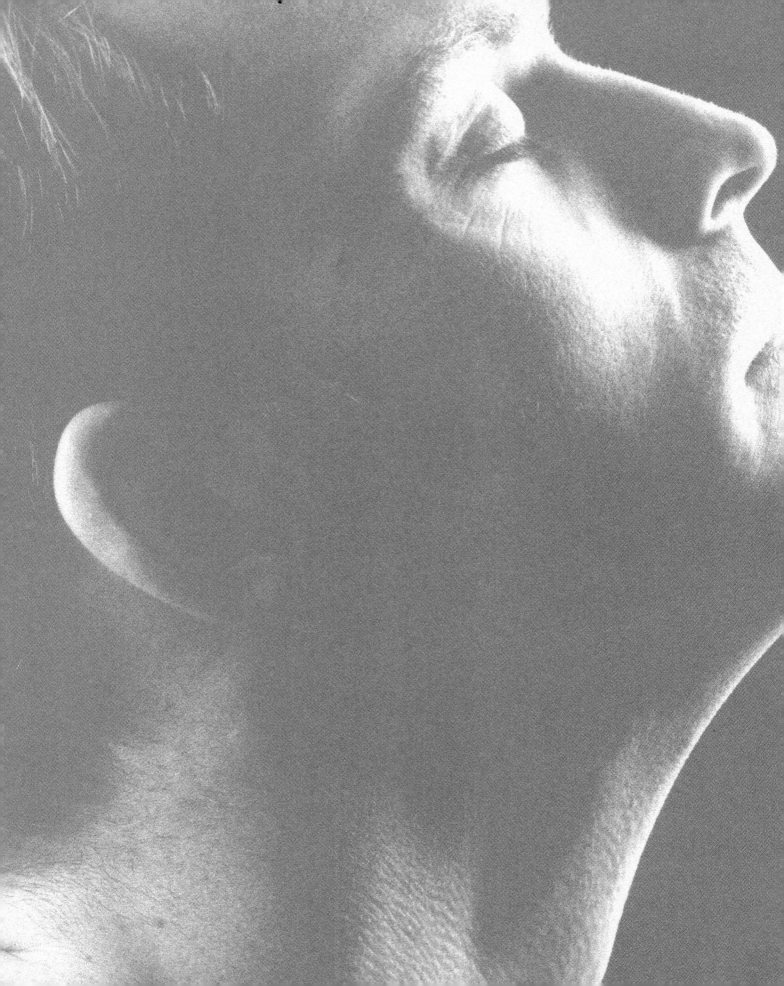

an introduction to
AROMATHERAPY

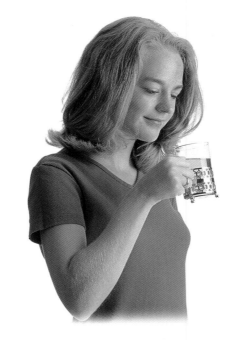

Nicola Jenkins

This is a Parragon Publishing book
First published in 2002

Parragon Publishing
Queen Street House
4 Queen Street
Bath, BA1 1HE, UK

This book was created by
THE BRIDGEWATER BOOK COMPANY

Art Director: Stephen Knowlden
Designers: Chris and Jane Lanaway
Editorial Director: Fiona Biggs
Project Editor: Lizzy Gray
Picture Researchers: Trudi Valter and Vanessa Fletcher
Photography: Ian Parsons

1-84273-439-3

Manufactured in China

DEDICATION
*This is for my mother, Carola Jenkins, and for
all my students—past and present*

Contents

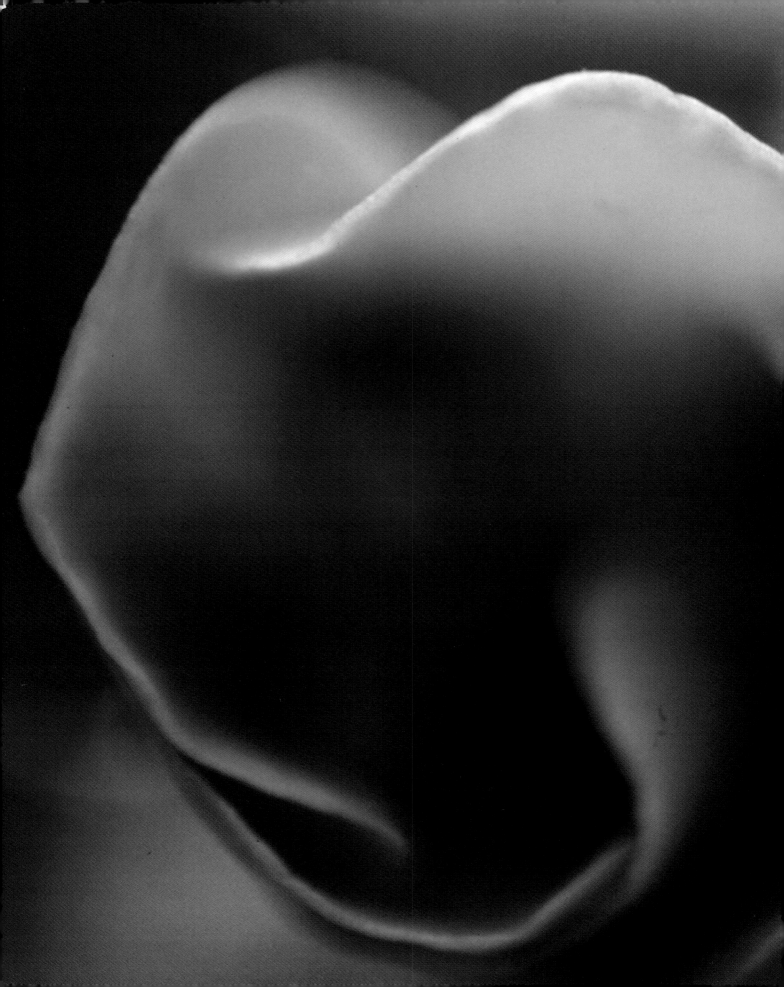

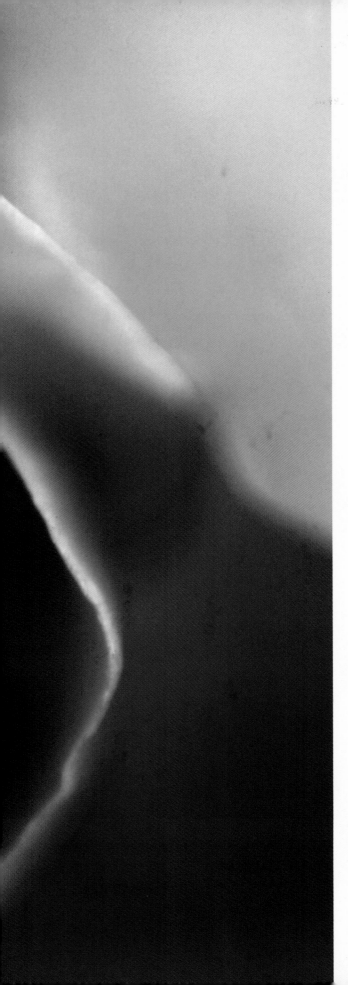

Introducing
aromatherapy

The first time you open a bottle of essential oil

is the moment in which you embark on an

adventure that can captivate all your senses—

one that might well occupy the rest of your life.

They can lift your spirits or calm you down,

removing all the cares and worries of your day.

Suddenly things won't feel quite so ordinary—

so breathe deeply.

What is aromatherapy?

Each day, every one of us comes into contact with some aspect of aromatherapy, whether we are aware of it or not. Divide the word "aromatherapy" in half, and you have "aroma"—meaning fragrance and "therapy"—meaning curative power or the encouragement of good health. There are certain aromas that we all associate with good health or well-being and cleanliness. They appear in our soaps, shampoos, cosmetics, and cleaning products and even in our food. Many companies, especially those in the Far East, are now piping essential oils through their buildings in order to keep employees healthy and happy or even to encourage customers to purchase their products.

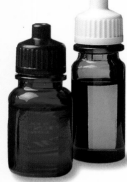

ESSENTIAL OIL
BOTTLES

When talking about aromatherapy as a form of therapy, most people associate it with massage. Massage is a key method of applying aromatherapy, but it is not the only way. Any method that involves applying essential oils in order to encourage good health or well-being is, by definition, a form of aromatherapy. You can practice aromatherapy in your car (prevent road rage with a tissue impregnated with essential oils), in your bath (add oils to your bath water), in your kitchen (use oils to enhance household cleaning) or in your bedroom (encourage restful sleep by using a vaporizer).

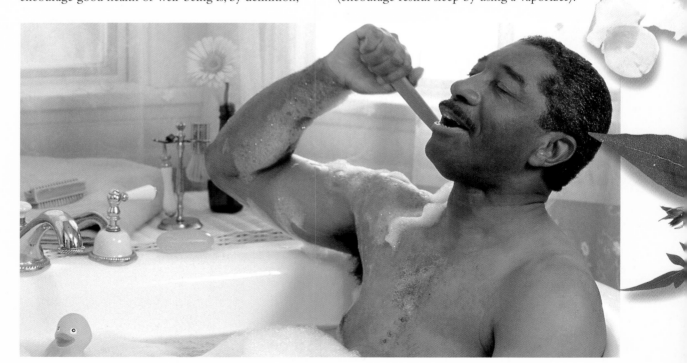

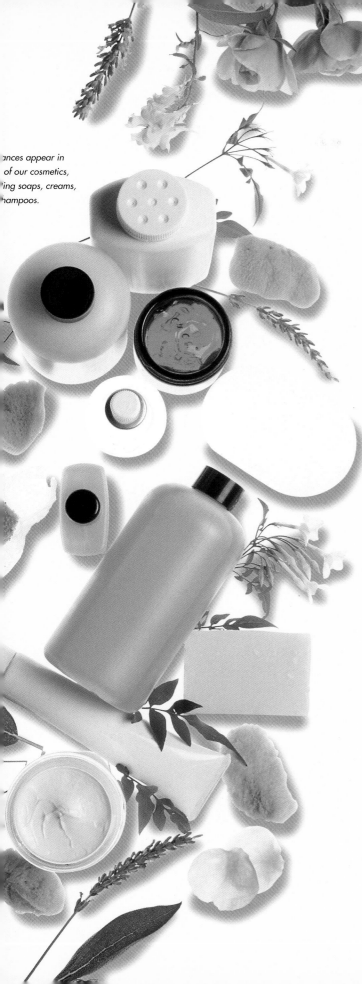

...ances appear in ... of our cosmetics, ...ing soaps, creams, ...hampoos.

ESSENTIAL OILS

Essential oils are at the core of the practice of aromatherapy. These highly fragrant and concentrated compounds are not actually "oils" at all, although they can dissolve in vegetable oils. Essential oils are extracted from various parts of plants—the roots, leaves, flowers, resin, bark, or even the peel of the fruit—through a number of methods, the most common of which is distillation. During distillation, steam is passed over plant parts in a still, then the steam passes into a condenser, where it produces a liquid containing both oil and water. The oil is then separated from the water. Extraction concentrates the potent liquids until the end product, the essence of the plant, is poured into a small bottle.

The extraction process varies with the essential oil being produced and, unfortunately, the price of the essential oil is a good guide to the difficulty involved in obtaining it. With essential oils, you really do get what you pay for. Expensive essential oils, such as jasmine, rose, or neroli, are very difficult to extract because it takes a large number of flowers to produce a small amount of essential oil. The price of essential oils can also vary with the weather and the geographical location of the crop—a poor harvest, soil low in nutrients, or a lack of sunlight that year are all contributing factors, which can lead to the production of less than satisfactory essential oils.

Most essential oils have a shelf-life of around two years after they have been extracted. The exceptions to this rule are the citrus oils—orange, lemon, lime, grapefruit, mandarin—as well as tagetes and angelica. In these cases, a six-month shelf-life is more likely. You can extend the shelf-life of your essential oils by storing them in a cool, dark place, such as the refrigerator, where they are not subject to sudden changes in temperature. If you do choose to store your essential oils in the refrigerator, keep them in an airtight container to prevent them from adding unexpected flavors to your food.

ROSE PETALS

Aromatherapy
through the ages

Humans have been harnessing the therapeutic, culinary, and fragrant effects of plants since before we came out of the caves. The incredible power of some of the plant compounds was believed to border on the magical; plants and resins such as Roman camomile, frankincense, benzoin, myrrh, cypress, jasmine, and rose made the leap into religious and ceremonial usage and our awareness and reverence for them have increased with time.

Juniper berries are not just used to flavor food: their essential oil is valued medicinally too.

AROMATHERAPY IN ANCIENT TIMES

Modern aromatherapy can trace its roots as far back as prehistoric times, when juniper was used as an antiseptic and to flavor food. As the centuries marched on, the use of plants for therapeutic reasons was documented in all the major civilizations. Sages in ancient China and India, for example, described the therapeutic properties of plants such as black pepper, which was used both as a febrifuge and a sudorific (to promote sweating).

The ancient Egyptians developed a complicated series of cosmetics, perfumes, incense, and embalming methods, which formed a central feature of civilized behavior in their society. Studies in Egyptian hieroglyphics have been instrumental in uncovering a great deal of information about the use of plant products for health and beauty at the time.

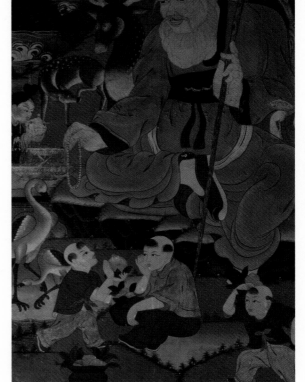

Sages in ancient India and China used the aromatic and healing properties of plants.

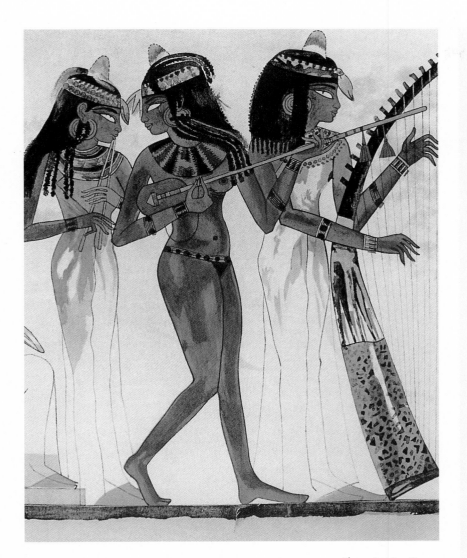

KYPHI INCENSE

Recapture some of the fragrances that drifted down the Nile in ancient Egypt. Creating the original Kyphi incense that scented the ancient temples would involve many days of careful preparation. This blend, for use in a vaporizer, includes many of the original ingredients. Prepare the blend in an amber glass bottle in advance. When ready to use, put 4–6 drops of the blend in the vaporizer:

INGREDIENTS

Lemongrass 4 drops
Cardamom 4 drops
Spikenard 4 drops
Juniper 8 drops
Marjoram 4 drops
Frankincense 15 drops
Myrrh 15 drops

The level of expertise in the use of plants appears to have reached a height during the reign of the female Pharaoh Hatshepsut, when Egypt started to grow some of the key ingredients of its cosmetics and incenses instead of continuing to import them. At this time, around 1500 BCE, one of the favorite cosmetics available to wealthier Egyptians was an unguent cone, which was made of fats and oils scented with fragrant plant materials, such as marjoram, myrrh, frankincense, or jasmine. Traces of other plants, such as Roman camomile, rosemary, or cedar, were also found in the wrappings of mummies: they were used as part of the embalming process, helping to keep people looking as young and well preserved in death as they did in life.

The ancient Egyptians used a variety of fragrant plants in their cosmetics and rituals, and also in their embalming process.

Fragrant and therapeutic plants were so sought-after that the incense and spice trades began to expand as early as 500 BCE. Countries that were rich in the desired plants began to increase dramatically in wealth and power, while conquering kings started to demand fragrant resins, such as frankincense, benzoin, and myrrh, in tribute. Indeed, they regarded these so highly that in some cases the resins were considered to be more valuable than gold and jewels.

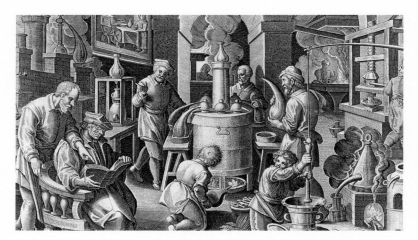

By the sixteenth century, knowledge of the distillation process and uses of essential oils was widespread in Europe.

MEDIEVAL AND MODERN AROMATHERAPY

Regardless of the wide range of therapeutic applications of the plants from which essential oils are derived, it wasn't until the process of distillation was discovered (or rediscovered) by Persian physician Avicenna around 1030 CE, that essential oils began to be prepared and used in a manner similar to that used today. Avicenna used distillation to extract essential oils from the rose, a notoriously difficult process, because you need a vast amount of roses to produce the essential oil in any reasonable quantity. From distilling roses, it was only a small step to distilling other plant products for their therapeutic and cosmetic properties. By 1597, when Jerome of Brunswick published *New Vollkomen Distillierbuch*, the understanding of distillation and the use of essential oils had become so widespread in Europe that he makes detailed references to over 20 essential oils, including

Persian physician and philosopher Avicenna (980–1037 CE) first distilled essential oil from roses. It is a difficult process that needs a large quantity of flowers.

lavender, clove, cinnamon, and rosemary. English physician Nicholas Culpeper also added significantly to our understanding of the properties of essential oils and plant remedies with the publication of his famous herbal in 1649.

Despite this long tradition of plant and herbal remedies and the history of empirical evidence of the effectiveness of essential oils, their use in allopathic or Western medicine has been rather limited. It was not until French perfumer and chemist René Gattefossé accidentally burned his hand in his laboratory in 1910 that the foundations of the current practice of aromatherapy began to develop. Gattefossé, in a great deal of pain, immediately stuck his hand in a nearby vat of lavender essential oil, which he mistook for water. When there was no swelling, pain, or blistering after what was expected to be a serious burn, he began the series of investigations and observations that were to establish this popular therapy. Gattefossé used essential oils in the treatment of soldiers' wounds during World War I, and his interests and results encouraged others to follow suit, among them Dr Jean Valnet. Valnet's work during and after the Indochina war (1948–1959) provided significant and comprehensive information on the effects of a range of essential oils on different medical conditions.

It took another biochemist, an Austrian called Marguerite Maury, to link the use of essential oils to cosmetics and massage, using carrier oils to dilute the essential oils appropriately. Maury's seminal text, *The Secret of Life and Youth*, alongside that of Robert Tisserand's *The Art of Aromatherapy*—the first book written and published in English on this subject—helped to establish the fundamental principles that holistic aromatherapists use today.

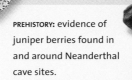
BLACK PEPPER

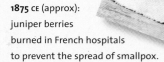
VICTORIAN BRIDAL HEADDRESS

NOTABLE EVENTS

PREHISTORY: evidence of juniper berries found in and around Neanderthal cave sites.

2000 BCE: black pepper described for its medicinal properties in ancient Chinese and Sanskrit texts; monks using black pepper to assuage hunger on long journeys.

JUNIPER BERRIES

1500 BCE: atlas, cedarwood, frankincense, cypress, and myrrh used by ancient Egyptians for embalming, religious rites, cosmetics, and perfumery, and in a blend as an antidote for poisoning.

776 BCE: Greece starts to use essential oils in water for floral fragrances, particularly orange, neroli, and lemon. Bay distillations and incense used by the Oracle at Delphi to induce prophecy.

496 BCE: frankincense taken as tribute by kings such as Nebuchadnezzar of Babylon and Darius of Persia—valued weight for weight with gold.

400 BCE: Greek physician Hippocrates uses camomile as a febrifuge (a medicine that reduces fever) and recommends daily massage with aromatic herbs for general good health.

226 BCE: courtiers advised to hold clove buds in their mouths to ensure sweet breath when addressing the Chinese emperor.

165 CE: Greek physician Galen recommends the use of cypress to ease diarrhea.

500–600 CE: India uses sandalwood-based incense for exorcism rites and for healing arrow wounds.

1000 CE: China imports frankincense for medicinal purposes.

1030 CE (approx): Persian physician Avicenna rediscovered the distillation process, and began distilling roses for the essential oil and flower water.

1400 CE: England starts to use herbal and infused oils for medicinal properties; frankincense and benzoin used to make Friar's Balsam for respiratory complaints and skin conditions.

1550 CE: (approx): Chinese physicians use sandalwood to treat cholera.

1600 CE: bergamot used in Italian folk medicine.

1649 CE: English physician Nicholas Culpeper publishes his herbal, which goes on to become a standard reference work for plant remedies.

1700 CE: eau de Cologne invented using rosemary, bergamot, neroli, lavender essential oils.

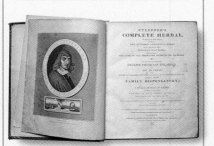
CULPEPER'S HERBAL

1800 CE: neroli used as a perfume by prostitutes in Madrid to help identify their profession.

1850 CE: neroli used in bridal headdresses in Victorian England to represent purity and virginity.

1875 CE (approx): juniper berries burned in French hospitals to prevent the spread of smallpox.

1922 CE: Tutankhamun's tomb opened—sealed bottles placed there at his incarceration in 1347–1339 BCE still retained their fragrance.

1910 CE: French chemist and perfumer, Gattefosé burns his hand in his laboratory, sticks it in a pot of essential oil of lavender, and rediscovers the healing properties of lavender.

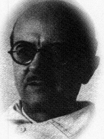
GATTEFFOSÉ

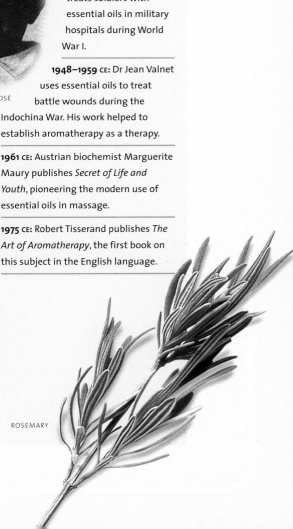
WORLD WAR I

1914–18 CE: Gattefossé treats soldiers with essential oils in military hospitals during World War I.

1948–1959 CE: Dr Jean Valnet uses essential oils to treat battle wounds during the Indochina War. His work helped to establish aromatherapy as a therapy.

1961 CE: Austrian biochemist Marguerite Maury publishes *Secret of Life and Youth*, pioneering the modern use of essential oils in massage.

1975 CE: Robert Tisserand publishes *The Art of Aromatherapy*, the first book on this subject in the English language.

ROSEMARY

Aromatherapy **today**

Aromatherapy is ideally suited to promote health and well-being and to reduce the effects of stress. That said, it is not intended to replace conventional medical treatment, but to complement it. If you are experiencing any symptoms that leave you worried or in prolonged pain, it is advisable to visit your doctor first.

Aromatherapists use essential oils in order to promote good health and well-being in their clients. If you visit an aromatherapist, you can expect to receive a massage as part of your treatment. While massage is not the only method of using essential oils, it is one of the most effective ways of administering them. As well as experiencing the beneficial effects of the massage, the time spent receiving the massage will let you relax and enjoy the beautiful fragrance created especially for you.

Aromatherapy is regarded as a "holistic" therapy, in that it takes into consideration the needs of the whole person. In other words, your visit to the aromatherapist will involve time spent discussing how you are feeling—not just physically, but mentally and emotionally too—in order to determine which essential oils are most appropriate for you at this time. There are always several essential oils that might be beneficial to you, and it is important that you help in the blending process by choosing the ones you like the most from the selection on offer. It is at this point that the creative fun begins! Blending the essential oils in various concentrations can create a whole palette of delightful fragrances to suit your needs, each with differing effects.

Aromatherapy is a holistic form of treatment, which means that it takes into account the needs of the whole person, physically, mentally, and emotionally.

HOW TO CREATE AN AROMATHERAPY BLEND

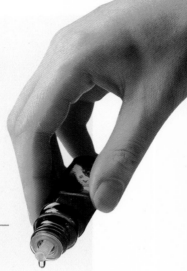

Check which essential oils are most appropriate for the person you are treating by reading the list of conditions each oil can help.

Make sure you are aware of any safety issues that could affect your treatment.

Let the person smell the oils you think are appropriate and choose their three favorites.

Follow the guidelines for the number of drops appropriate for each of the essential oils you have chosen. You do not have to use the full number of drops for each essential oil, but the total number of drops should not exceed eight for a healthy adult.

Create your blend by adding each drop slowly to the carrier oil or base product of your choice. A carrier oil, such as sunflower oil, sweet almond, or grapeseed oil, will provide a base for the essential oils without dispersing their active ingredients. See page 92.

If you accidentally add too many drops of essential oil, top up with additional carrier oil.

Mix well and leave in a dark container in a cool place until you are ready to use your blend.

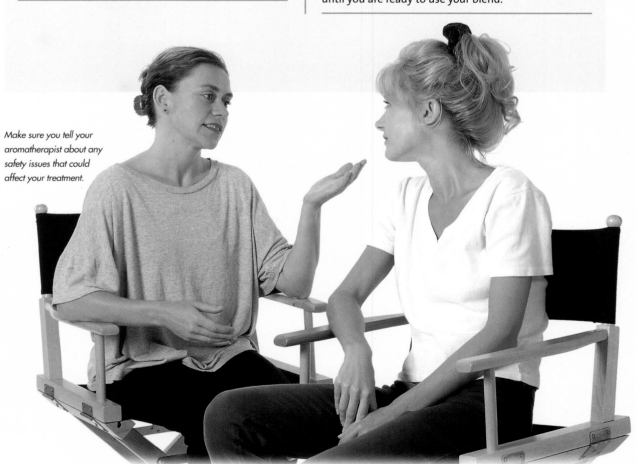

Make sure you tell your aromatherapist about any safety issues that could affect your treatment.

How aromatherapy **works**

Three aspects combine to make aromatherapy effective for promoting health and well-being. These are fragrance, chemicals, and massage.

Scents can be evocative, so a whiff of gingerbread, for example, could trigger a recollection of your grandmother's kitchen.

FRAGRANCE

Your sense of smell is the only sense that has nerve receptors exposed to the outside world. When these receptors pick up a fragrant "message," they transport it straight to the limbic system, deep within the brain, for processing and identification. The limbic system is also the place where memories are stored, which accounts in part for the reason that aromas are so evocative. For example, a whiff of ginger might transport you back to your grandmother's kitchen, or a hint of jasmine might make you remember a tropical beach. By creating a blend of essential oils that evoke pleasant memories, you can encourage relaxation, induce a sense of wellbeing and reduce stress and tension.

CHEMICALS

Each essential oil is made up of a large number of organic compounds, many of which have undergone laboratory testing and have been shown to have specific effects on the body's organs. In their natural state, as part of the essential oil, these chemical constituents work in harmony with each other and with the human body, and are generally free from the unpleasant side effects that can sometimes arise from using the isolated chemical, or so-called "active ingredient." When the essential oil is dissolved in a carrier oil (see pages 92–3) and spread over the body as part of a massage, the essential oil can make its way through the skin, enter the blood, and be transported

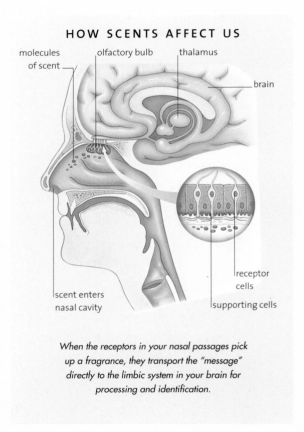

HOW SCENTS AFFECT US

molecules of scent

olfactory bulb

thalamus

brain

receptor cells

supporting cells

scent enters nasal cavity

When the receptors in your nasal passages pick up a fragrance, they transport the "message" directly to the limbic system in your brain for processing and identification.

around the body and to the brain. This is not dangerous because the essential oil is used at a very low dose in the massage and much of it will evaporate before entering the skin. Once in the body, the essential oils can start to work on a chemical level, including mimicking hormones, reducing muscle spasms, and relieving pain. Essential oils applied as part of a massage take about 20 minutes to get into the bloodstream, and in some cases their effects can last for about three days.

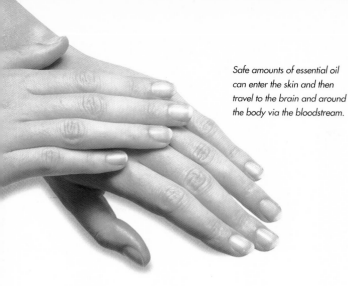

Safe amounts of essential oil can enter the skin and then travel to the brain and around the body via the bloodstream.

THE CIRCULATORY SYSTEM

lungs

heart

vein

artery

Massage with essential oils can improve the circulation of the blood and the lymphatic system, and reduce blood pressure.

MASSAGE

Massage is the most common method of applying aromatherapy as part of a treatment, and has distinct benefits for the person receiving it. Massage can improve the circulation of blood and lymph, reduce blood pressure, relieve pain, and lower the heart rate. Using essential oils increases the effects of the massage, and therapists sometimes claim that they are able to achieve in one aromatherapy treatment what they would expect to accomplish in four or five massages using carrier oil alone.

CHOOSING THE RIGHT ESSENTIAL OILS

It is important to understand the structure and functions of the various body systems, as well as the underlying causes of the discomfort experienced, in order to choose the best essential oils to use. For example, if you are experiencing a headache, understanding what is involved in the different types of headaches— migraines, tension headaches, or hangovers—will help you to make a more informed choice. For example, you might decide to use lavender on a cool compress for the migraine, Roman camomile and a back massage for the tension headache, or juniper in bath water (and a very large glass of water to drink) for the hangover.

You do not have to be suffering from an ailment to feel the benefits of aromatherapy —you can use essential oils to help promote relaxation and maintain good health too.

> **NOTE**
> For details of a wider range of essential oils, consult *An Introduction to Essential Oils* by Sara Rose, also in this series.

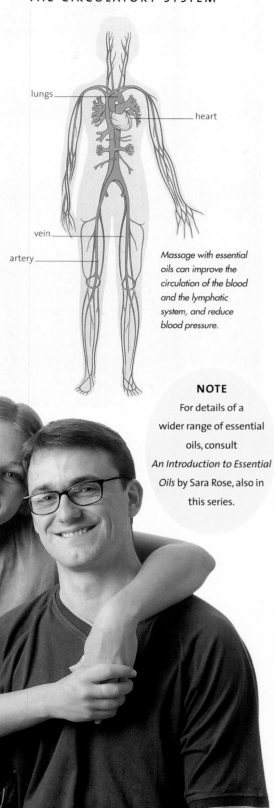

The **benefits** of aromatherapy

Throughout this book, you will find examples of essential oils that have been used with some success by qualified, practicing aromatherapists to treat a range of different conditions.

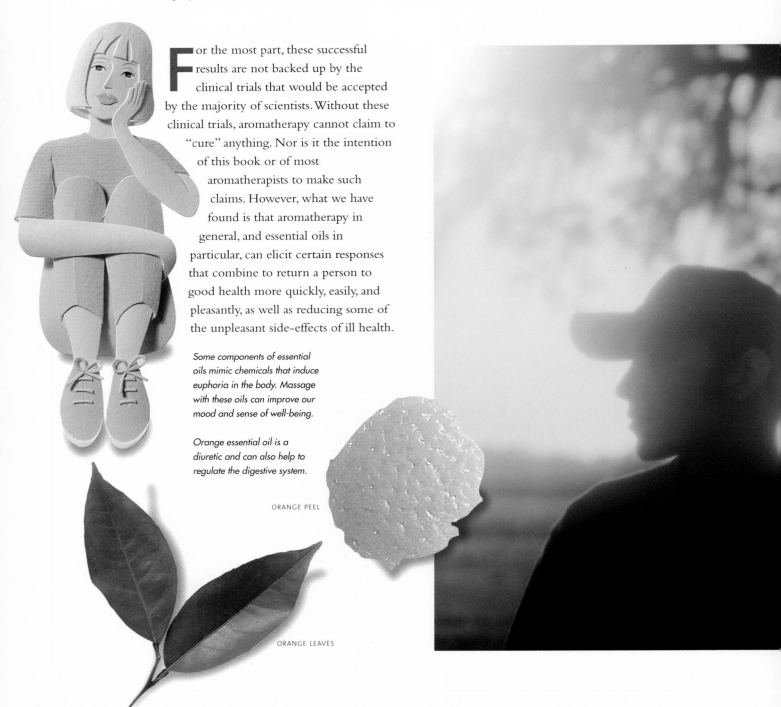

For the most part, these successful results are not backed up by the clinical trials that would be accepted by the majority of scientists. Without these clinical trials, aromatherapy cannot claim to "cure" anything. Nor is it the intention of this book or of most aromatherapists to make such claims. However, what we have found is that aromatherapy in general, and essential oils in particular, can elicit certain responses that combine to return a person to good health more quickly, easily, and pleasantly, as well as reducing some of the unpleasant side-effects of ill health.

Some components of essential oils mimic chemicals that induce euphoria in the body. Massage with these oils can improve our mood and sense of well-being.

Orange essential oil is a diuretic and can also help to regulate the digestive system.

ORANGE PEEL

ORANGE LEAVES

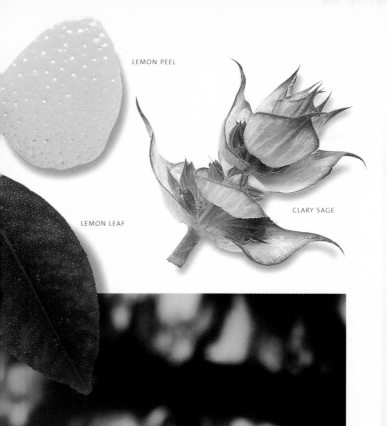

LEMON PEEL

LEMON LEAF

CLARY SAGE

AROMATHERAPY CAN

Improve mood and general feeling of well-being—both through relaxing massage and through the use of essential oils where the components mimic certain euphoria-inducing chemicals that are present in the body.

Improve blood and lymphatic circulation through massage and the use of essential oils that contain chemicals able to constrict or dilate blood vessels and raise or lower blood pressure.

Encourage the endocrine system to balance hormone production and dispersal. A number of essential oils contain chemicals that are structurally similar to certain hormones or can mimic their effects. Clary sage and fennel, for instance, can mimic the action of estrogen.

Improve digestion by relieving cramps, bowel spasms, and bloating.

Aid the immune system by killing bacterial and fungal infections.

Slow down excessive production of waste products, such as sweat, diarrhea, and menstrual blood.

Increase production of urine through the diuretic properties of a number of essential oils, including juniper, grapefruit, lemon, and orange.

Reduce pain and encourage restful sleep. Many essential oils contain chemicals that have been used to produce strong pain-killers, antispasmodics, and sedatives—Valium, for instance, is derived from valerian essential oil.

FENNEL

Using aromatherapy safely

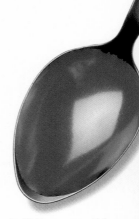

It takes over 10,000 lemons to make 2 teaspoons/10 ml of lemon essential oil. These highly concentrated, aromatic liquids may smell like bottled sunlight but, just like sunlight, we have to be careful about how we use them. Remember that less is more—you do not have to use the maximum number of drops suggested for each essential oil. Instead, try blending them in different proportions to achieve spectacular results.

To fill this teaspoon with lemon essential oil, you would need 5,000 lemons. This is why some essential oils can be expensive.

BLENDING

When you start blending, you should stick to two simple rules:

1 For a healthy adult, essential oils should comprise 2% or less of a solution (that means a total of 8 drops of essential oil per 4 teaspoons/20 ml of carrier oil (see page 92–3) or 20 drops per 1¾ oz/50 g of moisturizing cream).

2 Stick to three essential oils or fewer in each blend, at least until you feel confident of your blending.

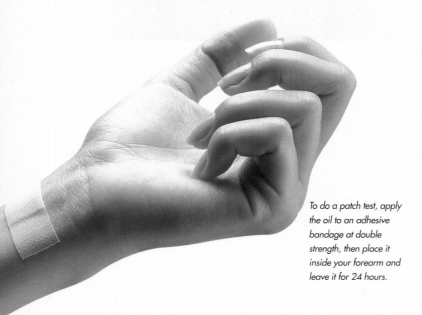

To do a patch test, apply the oil to an adhesive bandage at double strength, then place it inside your forearm and leave it for 24 hours.

PATCH TESTING

If you suspect you may be sensitive to an essential oil or carrier oil (see page 92–3), do a patch test first. Apply the oil to an adhesive bandage at double the concentration you want to use. Place the bandage on the inside of your forearm and leave it in place for 24 hours. If you experience no reaction, the oil is safe for you to use. People with an allergy to citrus fruit might wish to patch test the essential oils extracted from citrus peel, including orange, lemon, grapefruit, lime, bergamot, and mandarin. Neroli and petitgrain are also products of citrus plants, but are unlikely to cause an adverse reaction. Other essential oils that can sometimes affect sensitive skin are lemongrass, melissa, may chang, eucalyptus, and jasmine.

ADVERSE REACTION

If you have an adverse reaction—anything from itchiness to raised red blotches—wash the skin quickly and thoroughly with unperfumed soap. Expose the affected skin to the air to encourage the essential oils to evaporate. Essential oils of yarrow, German camomile and lavender all help to reduce inflammation and stop itchiness. Have these oils at hand in a lotion or cream, especially if you suspect an adverse reaction may occur. Essential oils in the correct dose should not cause an irritation, but this is a possibility in cases of very sensitive skin.

USING ESSENTIAL OILS SAFELY

Keep essential oils out of the reach of children.

Do not apply essential oils to open wounds.

If you have sensitive skin or suspect an allergy, carry out a patch test prior to using the essential oils (see page 20).

Contact a doctor immediately if you suffer any adverse reaction.

Avoid using sunbeds or going out in bright sunlight for 12 hours after using citrus oils.

Do not take essential oils by mouth.

Keep essential oils away from your eyes.

Reduce the amount of essential oil by at least half for women who are pregnant, children between 2 and 12 years of age, the elderly, and people with sensitive skin.

Children up to the age of 2 years should not receive more than 2 drops of essential oil in 100 ml/3½ fl oz of carrier oil.

Avoid using essential oils on the skin during the first three months of pregnancy, especially if you have a history of miscarriages or unstable pregnancies.

Avoid using tea tree and rosemary oils at any time during pregnancy.

The following oils are safe to use in very small quantities during the latter stages of pregnancy: neroli, lavender, Roman camomile, German camomile, geranium, patchouli, petitgrain, and sandalwood.

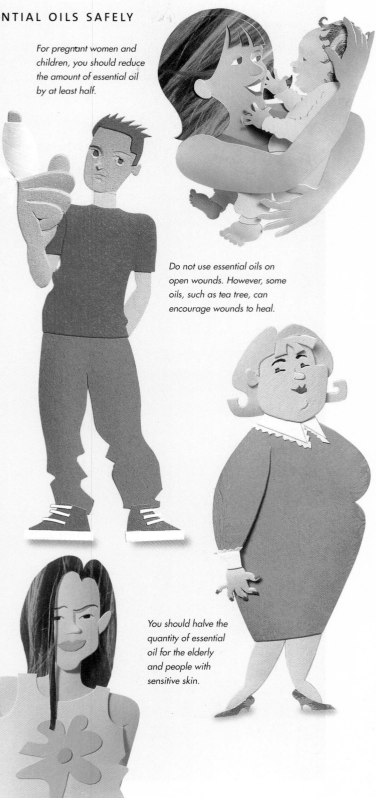

For pregnant women and children, you should reduce the amount of essential oil by at least half.

Do not use essential oils on open wounds. However, some oils, such as tea tree, can encourage wounds to heal.

You should halve the quantity of essential oil for the elderly and people with sensitive skin.

If you have been using citrus oils, you should avoid using a sunbed or going out in bright sunshine for at least 12 hours afterward.

How to use essential oils

Most essential oils are created by distilling tonnes of plant material. These tiny bottles of oil are highly concentrated in their final form, so they need to be handled with care if you are going to avoid an unpleasant reaction. Always remember to dilute the essential oils appropriately for the person you are treating. The guidelines below are suitable for a healthy adult. If you are treating someone who is either pregnant or under 12 years of age, or who has sensitive, diseased, or damaged skin, you will need to alter the amount of essential oils used in any method that puts these in direct contact with the skin, such as bathing, bath products, moisturizers and massage oils. See page 12 for details.

BATH

Add a maximum of 4–6 drops of essential oils to a deep bath (for an adult only). To encourage relaxation, and to relieve muscular aches and pains, painful joints, painful periods, and cystitis, try cedarwood, geranium, lavender, rose, and sandalwood.

Keep citrus, lemongrass, and rosemary oils to a minimum—less than 2 drops in a deep bath. These oils can sometimes irritate the skin when used in this fashion.

HOUSEHOLD CLEANING

Add 3–4 drops of essential oil to a bucket of soapy water for wiping down surfaces or mopping floors—it can be used daily. Essential oils that are particularly known for their anti-bacterial properties include all citrus oils, lavender, niaouli, pine, silver fir, and tea tree.

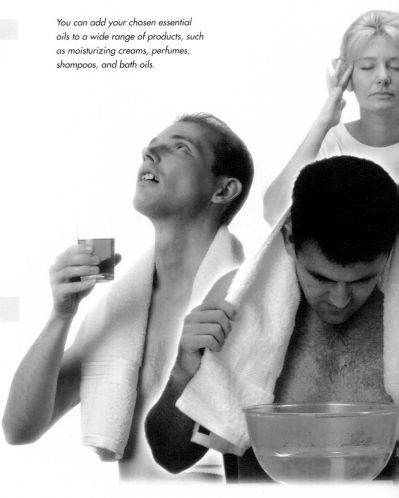

You can add your chosen essential oils to a wide range of products, such as moisturizing creams, perfumes, shampoos, and bath oils.

MOISTURIZER

Mix 20 drops of essential oil in 1¾ oz/50 g of cream base. Useful for many skin conditions, but particularly helpful for dry or aging skin or eczema. Try cedarwood, frankincense, geranium, neroli, patchouli, rose, sandalwood, and vetiver.

INHALATIONS

Add 4–6 drops to a bowl of steaming hot water, then hold your head over the basin and place a towel over your head. Try frankincense, benzoin, cedarwood, naouli, pine, and sandalwood.

INHALATIONS FOR COUGHS, COLDS, AND BRONCHITIS

This method can also be used to steam the face because it will open pores prior to an extended beauty treatment. Try essential oils that help the respiratory system to function efficiently, or that stimulate the immune system, such as benzoin, bergamot, cedarwood, frankincense, lavender, lemon, marjoram, melissa, orange, or sandalwood.

PERFUME

Add 12 drops of essential oil to 2¾fl oz/80 ml of equal parts rosewater and alcohol. This can be used at any time! Remember to shake the perfume well before applying. Try bergamot, grapefruit, jasmine, neroli, patchouli, rose, sandalwood, vetiver, and ylang ylang.

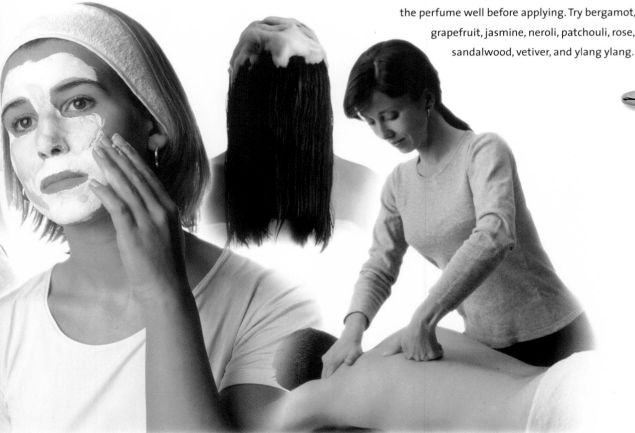

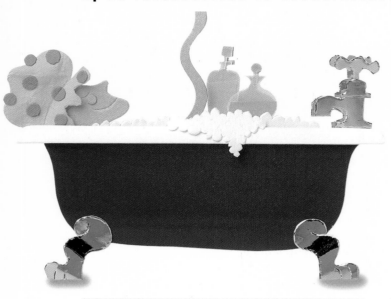

Adding eight drops of your chosen essential oil to your bubble bath base will make bathtimes very relaxing.

SHOWER GEL

Add 10 drops of essential oil to 1 fl oz/30 ml of shower gel base. Useful for easing skin conditions such as stress-related eczema, or respiratory conditions where there is no time or inclination to bathe. Use benzoin, cedarwood, frankincense, grapefruit, lavender, lemon, may chang, palmarosa, peppermint, rosemary, and yarrow.

BUBBLE BATH

Mix 8 drops of essential oil with 4 teaspoons/ 20 ml of bubble bath base, then add to a deep bath. This is a useful method of diluting essential oils for use on sensitive skin. Use cedarwood, geranium, grapefruit, jasmine, lavender, lemon, marjoram, orange rose, rosewood, sandalwood, or yarrow.

ROOM FRAGRANCER

Mix 10–15 drops of essential oil with cold water and then pour into a plant spray. Shake before use and spray around the room. This spray can be used daily, and is useful for supporting the immune system and easing respiratory conditions. Use cinnamon, frankincense, grapefruit, juniper, lemon, and rosemary.

Add 10–15 drops of essential oil to a plant spray filled with cold water and spray around a room to give it an uplifting and healing atmosphere.

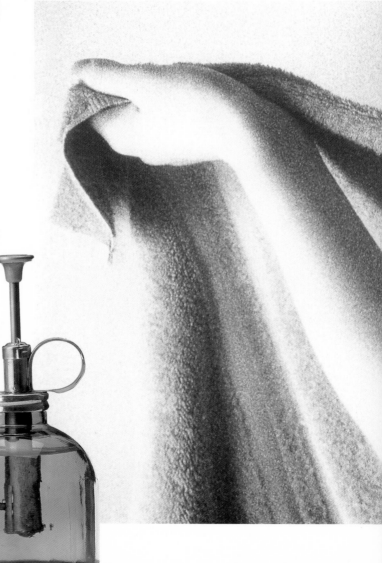

MASSAGE OIL

To make a massage oil, add 8 drops of essential oil to 4 teaspoons/20 ml of a carrier oil such as grapeseed (see pages 92–3 for more details of appropriate carrier oils). This is a good, general purpose way to treat most mild conditions—the most common method of using essential oils as part of an aromatherapy treatment. Try vetiver, geranium, jasmine, lavender, lemon, marjoram, patchouli, rose, and sandalwood.

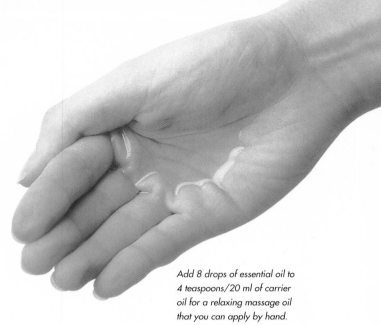

Add 8 drops of essential oil to 4 teaspoons/20 ml of carrier oil for a relaxing massage oil that you can apply by hand.

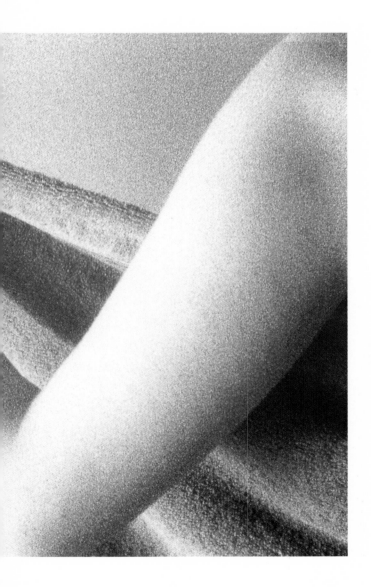

ESSENTIAL OIL VAPORIZER

Use 5 drops of essential oil to fragrance a room, aid sleep (do not leave candles burning unattended), ease coughing or breathing difficulties, calm the mind, or stimulate the immune system. All essential oils can be used in this way. Try black pepper, clary sage, cedarwood, citrus oils, frankincense, juniper, lavender, lemongrass, marjoram, myrrh, peppermint, rosemary, and rosewood.

SHAMPOO

Mix 8 drops of essential oil with 4 teaspoons/ 20 ml of shampoo base, then use the shampoo as normal. For all hair and scalp conditions, you can also use peppermint or rosemary to increase circulation of blood to the scalp, particularly in cases of dandruff or hair loss. Try bergamot, cedarwood, grapefruit, lavender, lemon, peppermint, Roman camomile, rosemary, rosewood, tea tree, or yarrow.

Aromatherapy and **first aid**

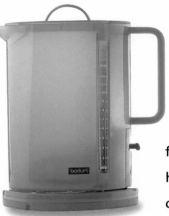

Soothe the pain of a minor burn from scalding water by putting a drop of neat essential oil directly on the affected part.

Aromatherapy can provide essential first-aid support for a wide variety of minor conditions, such as cuts, scrapes, scalds, sunburn, and insect bites and stings. Remember René Gatteffosé's experiences in his laboratory (see page 12) and keep a bottle of lavender in the kitchen, for use as a modern first-aid remedy. No kitchen should be without one! Minor burns from hot dishes, scalding water, or an iron can be treated quickly with a drop of the neat essential oil placed immediately over the burn. This can help to reduce or prevent blistering and will relieve pain. Tea tree is another essential oil that is invaluable in an emergency and is particularly effective at healing insect bites and infections—a must for frequent travelers. Both lavender and tea tree essential oils can be used very effectively in hot and cold compresses to ease swelling, reduce pain, or to clean minor cuts and scrapes.

The kitchen is full of implements that can inflict minor injuries such as cuts and burns. Keep lavender and tea tree essential oils in the kitchen, just in case.

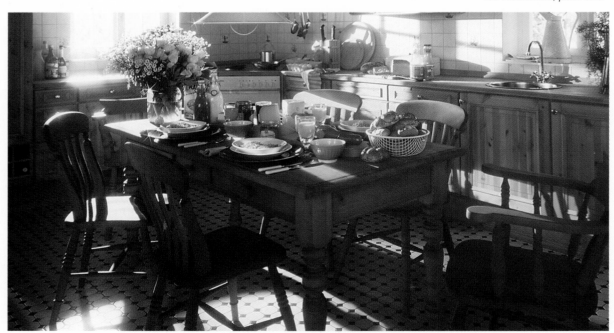

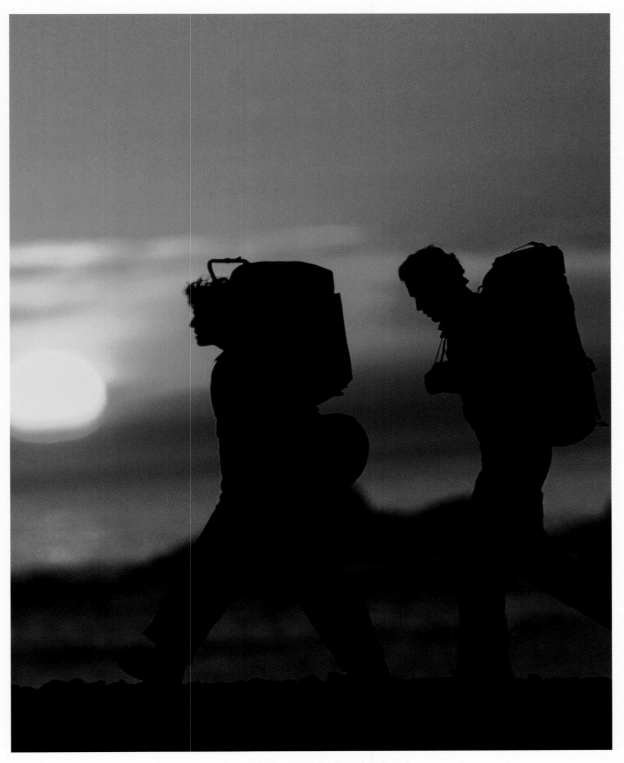

Essential oils can provide a host of soothing remedies for cuts, grazes, insect bites, and sunburn, so they are ideal for travelers.

Lavender Lavandula angustifolia

Lavender is the essential oil most people are introduced to first—and with good reason. The wide range of conditions it can help to ease make it a 'must-have' in any modern aromatherapy collection, just as it has been a major part of herb gardens since the middle ages. Those who love lavender might like to think about collecting samples of essential oils grown in different places; growing conditions can significantly alter the aroma.

Lavender essential oil is ideal for treating bruises—it will help to ease the discomfort and will also encourage healing.

SAFETY NOTE

unlikely to cause any adverse reactions

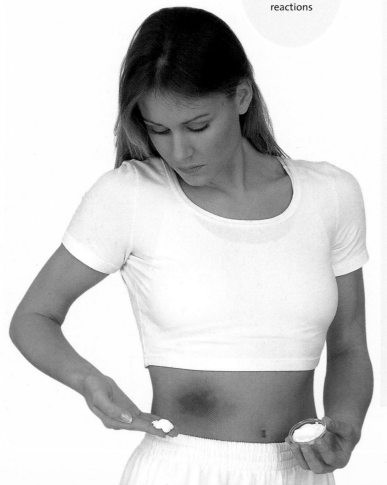

DATA FILE

GROWN IN: Europe—France, England, Bulgaria, Croatia

IN A BLEND: 4 drops in 4 teaspoons /20 ml carrier oil (see pages 92–3)

FOR THE BODY: relieves muscle spasms—especially in overworked muscles—as well as those caused by spastic colon, constipation, or irritable bowel; relieves itching from insect bites and stings as well as itching caused by eczema and dermatitis; reduces bacterial and fungal infections, thereby relieving conditions such as acne, cystitis, thrush, and athlete's foot; stimulates the immune system; relieves minor burns and heals wounds and bruising; helps to lower blood pressure; relieves pain related to headaches, migraines, endometriosis, and swollen breasts; eases breathing difficulties caused by asthma, and emphysema.

FOR THE MIND: aids in relieving anxiety, depression, insomnia, panic attacks, or cravings following the withdrawal of addictive substances (such as caffeine, nicotine or alcohol).

BLENDS WELL WITH: rosemary, marjoram, peppermint, neroli, rose, lemon, bergamot, sandalwood, geranium, Roman camomile, yarrow, melissa.

Tea tree oil is an excellent remedy for athlete's foot.

Tea tree Melaleuca alternifolia

Extensively used by Australian aboriginal tribes for its effectiveness in clearing infections, coughs, colds, and headaches. In particular, tea tree's ability to clear bacteria, now known worldwide, emerged when a Dr Penfold carried out research on the oil in 1923. He found it to be 12 times more effective at killing bacteria than the standard hospital disinfectant of the time—carbolic acid. For this reason, tea tree is also an increasingly popular component of shampoos, soaps, and cosmetics.

Tea tree oil is extracted from the leaves of the tree, which grows in Australia. Small branches are also used.

DATA FILE

GROWN IN: Australia

IN A BLEND: 3 drops in 4 teaspoons/20 ml of carrier oil

FOR THE BODY: helps to fight bacterial, viral and fungal infections such as acne, athlete's foot, cold sores, impetigo, nailbed infections, thrush, ringworm, verrucas, warts, and chicken pox; eases mild inflammatory conditions such as insect bites and stings, bronchitis, cystitis, and sinusitis. Tea tree is also an excellent supporting oil for the immune system, and helpful for people with post-viral fatigue or recurring glandular fever.

FOR THE MIND: helps to relieve lethargy, chronic anxiety, and poor concentration.

BLENDS WELL WITH: peppermint, bergamot, lavender, and eucalyptus.

Tea tree's antibacterial properties make it a popular ingredient in soaps, shampoos, and other cosmetics.

SAFETY NOTE
unlikely to cause any adverse reactions

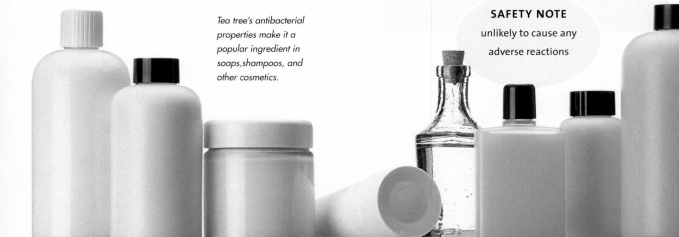

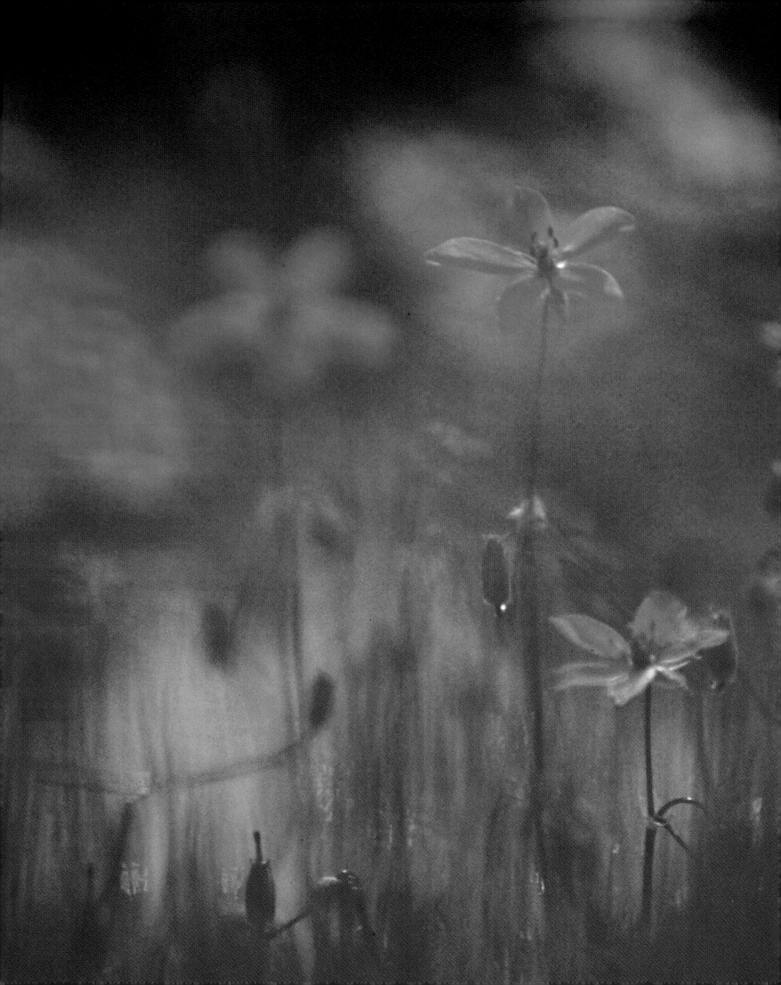

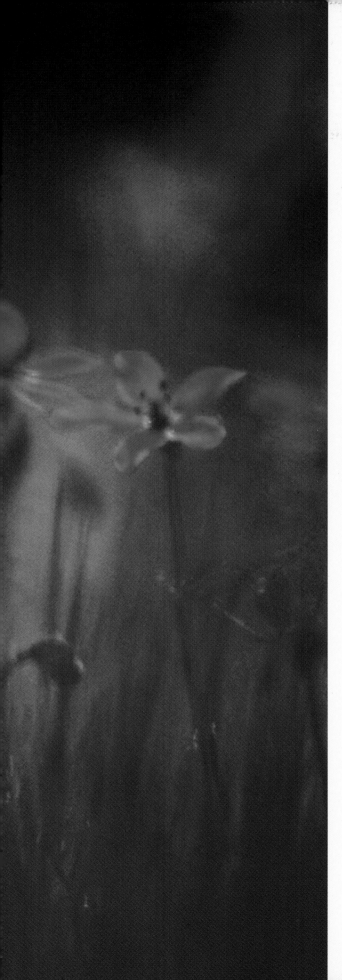

Practical
aromatherapy

Now is the time to get creative and find out just
how much these powerful, heavenly-scented
oils can improve your health. In the following
pages we look at how aromatherapy can be
used to ease the effects of stress on the different
body systems plus some simple massage
techniques you can use safely at home.

Aromatherapy for **stress relief**

The countless euphorics, sedatives, relaxants, and immune stimulants found in any collection of essential oils make up a formidable army when it comes to fighting the effects of stress. You will never be far from a practical solution to ease the symptoms you face when you employ the different oils and techniques covered here.

THE EFFECTS OF STRESS ON THE BODY

Your body is like a rubber band: you can stretch it to its limits physically and it will usually bounce back to its normal or resting state. However, if you keep stretching the rubber band, it will eventually either lose its ability to return to its normal size and shape or it will snap. The same thing can happen to the body when we put it under stress. A little stress is good for us: it keeps us fit and our minds active. Often it is accompanied by a feeling that we are working at the peak of our abilities.

Human bodies respond to stress by releasing chemicals that make our hearts beat faster, giving us the energy to carry out amazing feats of endurance, strength, or stamina, and causing blood and oxygen to race to the vital organs so that our minds feel clear—even at the point of crisis. Our bodies can deal with a lot of emergencies and our ability to leap into action (mental or physical) is part of what we call the "fight or flight" response.

However, too much stress, or a stressful situation that goes on for too long, can reduce your body's ability to work or rest effectively. Symptoms might start with depression, anxiety, irritability, or anger. They could move on to insomnia, headaches, migraines, exhaustion, indigestion, irritable bowel, menstrual difficulties, and much more serious conditions. Without due care, what may have started as a small hint from your body that it needs a holiday could eventually spiral out of control until you find yourself flat on your back for quite some time.

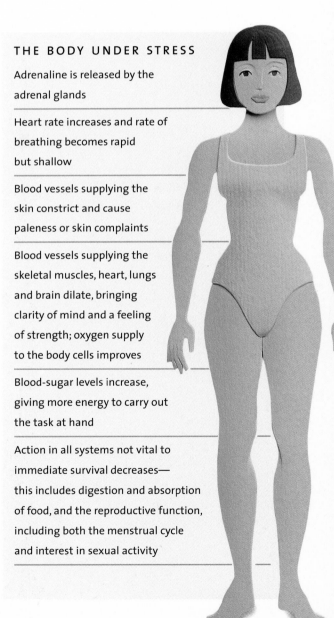

THE BODY UNDER STRESS

Adrenaline is released by the adrenal glands

Heart rate increases and rate of breathing becomes rapid but shallow

Blood vessels supplying the skin constrict and cause paleness or skin complaints

Blood vessels supplying the skeletal muscles, heart, lungs and brain dilate, bringing clarity of mind and a feeling of strength; oxygen supply to the body cells improves

Blood-sugar levels increase, giving more energy to carry out the task at hand

Action in all systems not vital to immediate survival decreases—this includes digestion and absorption of food, and the reproductive function, including both the menstrual cycle and interest in sexual activity

Each of us experiences stress in slightly different ways. Many people complain of tight muscles in necks and shoulders. Some note a change in the quality and clarity of their skin. Others experience digestive difficulties, thrush or cystitis, mood swings, poor quality of sleep, or a decrease in resistance to viruses such as the common cold or flu. If we pay attention to what our bodies are trying to tell us and give them time to recover, or reduce the things adding stress to our lives, we can function more effectively and much more happily.

TREATING STRESS

You can deal with stress in one of two ways: either treat the symptoms you are experiencing (for instance, start using peppermint oil in a massage blend to treat the bloating, constipation, and pain associated with irritable bowel) or treat the cause. If stress has reached a level in your life where you are experiencing unpleasant physical symptoms on a regular or prolonged basis, it is time to look seriously at treating both the symptoms and the cause and perhaps review your lifestyle.

Aromatherapy can help to improve your health and wellbeing, but without changes to your stressful lifestyle, it can only do so much. Lifestyle changes can be as big or as small as you like. Simple things like taking up a new hobby or meditation, reducing caffeine, nicotine, and alcohol intake, increasing the amount of plain water you drink, or indulging in a physical activity that you enjoy, can all help to improve the quality of your life and reduce stress in the process.

HOW MUCH STRESS ARE YOU UNDER?

The following items are just some of the things that contribute to the stress of modern living. Add a few of them together, and it is little wonder that we can begin to experience some of the physical symptoms of stress, disease, or emotional exhaustion.

Chemical/Environmental

Tea, coffee, caffeine, alcohol, nicotine, pesticides, herbicides, food intolerances (particularly dairy or wheat), noise pollution, noxious fumes, lead, asbestos, lack of sunlight, low air quality, high pollen count

Lifestyle

Moving house, change or loss of relationship, change or loss of job, financial worries, pregnancy, examinations, family members leaving home, change in sleeping habits, bereavement, personal injury

Making simple changes to your lifestyle, such as taking up meditation, can help reduce stress and improve the quality of your life.

Aromatherapy **massage** for the **face**

Use one drop of essential oil in 1 teaspoon/5 ml of carrier oil (see pages 92–93). With practice, this whole routine can take as little as 10 minutes, including cleansing and toning the skin prior to massage. To reduce fine lines substantially, why not incorporate this massage as part of your daily routine?

To carry out this massage as a treat for a friend, you can stretch the massage out to take up to 40 minutes. Simply repeat step 1 between each of the other steps and concentrate on the areas where most people find they are tense—at the jaw, the temples and over the forehead.

1 Effleurage the face, moving your hands from the chin along the jaw to the ears, then back to the chin, around the mouth and across the cheek bones to the temples, then back to the chin, around the mouth, up the sides of the nose, and across the forehead to the temples. Keep these movements rhythmic and gentle, remember that pressure is always up towards the forehead and towards the temples. Don't drag the skin downwards. Your friend should feel as if he or she has had a 'face lift' at the end of the treatment!

2 Use your thumb and index finger to squeeze the flesh along the jawline (imagine you are squeezing toothpaste out of a tube—pressure is towards the ear).

TIP
To perform effleurage, use gentle, stroking movements. The hands should glide smoothly over the skin.

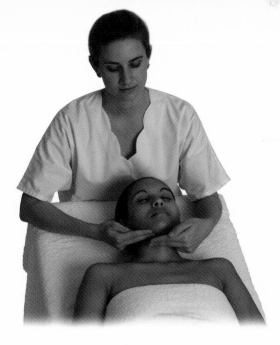

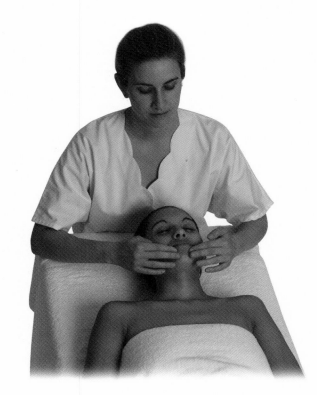

3 Using two fingers from each hand, pat along the jawline, then in lines across the face—from chin to temples, mouth to temples, nose to temples. This increases blood circulation to these areas and helps to tighten the underlying muscles.

4 Using your fingertips, stroke the skin in circular movements around the mouth. This is particularly good if you suffer from toothache or gum disease.

5 Using your fingertips, work in circles over the muscle just in front of each ear —where the jaw attaches to the skull. This is extremely effective if your friend grinds his or her teeth during sleep (or when angry!).

Aromatherapy **massage** for the **face**

6 Massage the ears with your fingertips.

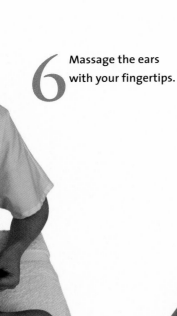

7 Using your index fingers, stroke up the sides of nose in circular movements: stroke up to the hairline and off the forehead.

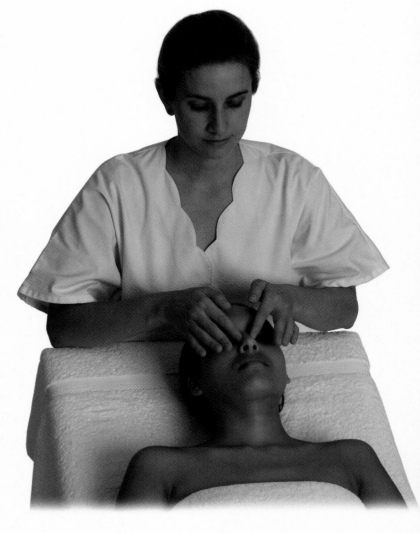

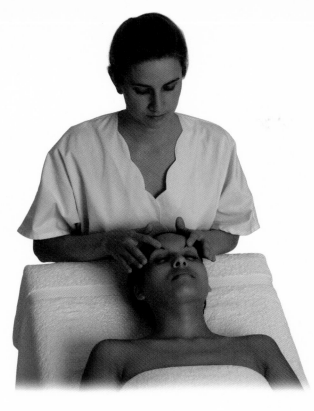

9 Trace your thumbs gently across the forehead from the center to the temples. Repeat this step several times.

8 Stroke above the eyes in circular movements, moving along the eyebrows to the temples. Rotate your fingers at the temples and then return very gently under the eyes (the skin under the eyes is particularly sensitive, so your fingers should hardly be touching the area) and back to the starting point. This can be very useful for reducing frown lines and easing painful sinusitis. Repeat this step five times.

10 Finish with your hands lightly cupped over the forehead. Run your fingers along the scalp and through the hair, then gently lift off your hands.

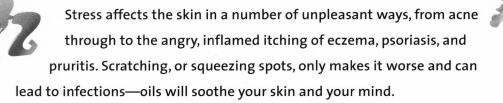

Lavender essential oil helps to combat infections and soothes itching skin.

Breaking out:
aromatherapy for the **skin**

Stress affects the skin in a number of unpleasant ways, from acne through to the angry, inflamed itching of eczema, psoriasis, and pruritis. Scratching, or squeezing spots, only makes it worse and can lead to infections—oils will soothe your skin and your mind.

The essential oils suggested here are all particularly effective at easing stress–related skin conditions. In the first instance, always turn to lavender or tea tree because these will combat infections as well as relieving the itching. Yarrow and both Roman and German camomile will help to reduce any swelling. However, you can also blend the oils to create a beautifully fragrant product that is a pleasure to wear all day or all night. Try jojoba as a carrier oil if you want to try a face oil: this will not only dissolve sebum (an oily substance) in blocked pores, but will help to reduce fine lines and can be used under makeup during the day. Stress-related skin conditions also respond particularly well when you increase the amount of water you drink. This encourages the body to work efficiently, and helps to remove toxins. For best results, aim to drink at least 4 pints/2 liters of water a day.

Try using jojoba as a carrier oil (see pages 92–3) to help clear blocked pores and reduce fine lines.

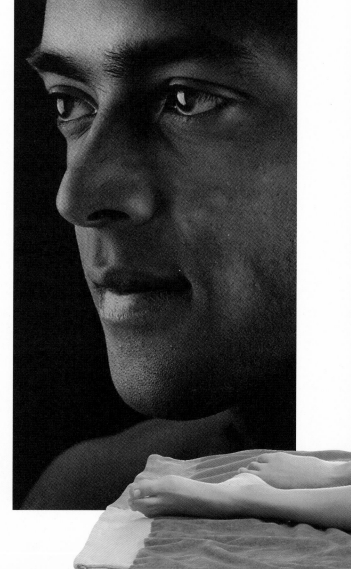

Benzoin, geranium, palmarosa, patchouli, rosewood, and sandalwood essential oils all help to balance and remoisturize dry skin.

DATA FILE

CONDITION	USEFUL ESSENTIAL OILS
Acne	Cedarwood, juniper, lavender, lemon, palmarosa, peppermint, rosemary, and tea tree
Eczema, dermatitis	Bergamot, cedarwood, geranium, German camomile, lavender, Roman camomile, sandalwood, and yarrow
Shingles or cold sores	Bergamot, cedarwood, geranium, lemon melissa, rose, tea tree
Fungal infections such as ringworm and athlete's foot	Lemon, manuka, niaouli, pine, and tea tree
Warts/verrucas	Lavender, lemon, manuka, niaouli, pine, and tea tree
Inflammation	Geranium, German camomile, lavender, rose, and yarrow
Burns, scalds, and sunburn	Cedarwood, German camomile, lavender, peppermint, tea tree, and yarrow
Bites and stings	Lavender, manuka, and tea tree
Oily skin	Bergamot, cypress, lemon, lemongrass, juniper, niaouli, tea tree, and rosemary
Stretch marks and scars	Frankincense, geranium, lavender, neroli, patchouli, rose, and rosewood
Dry skin	Benzoin, geranium, palmarosa, patchouli, rosewood, and sandalwood
Aging skin	Frankincense, lavender, neroli, palmarosa, and rose
Impetigo/pruritis	Geranium, German camomile, juniper, lavender, melissa, peppermint, rose, tea tree, and yarrow

Lavender and frankincense oils are good for stretchmarks from pregnancy.

Use lavender or German camomile essential oils to soothe inflamed or sunburned skin.

Fighting back: aromatherapy and the **immune** system

The immune system is responsible for helping us to fight infections and disease. It is your body's army, a collection of white blood cells, lymph nodes, and lymphatic tissue placed at strategic locations, all designed to fight the invading bacteria, viruses, fungi, and parasites that enter the body on a daily basis.

When infection occurs, symptoms can include fever, inflammation, an allergic reaction, and a variety of other symptoms related to the particular invading organism. Stress can reduce the effectiveness of the immune system, particularly if the individual feels that he or she lacks care, support, or understanding from close relatives or friends. The oils listed here are effective at helping to provide that support, but they are no substitute for it. Why not combine them with a simple back massage or take time out to relax and talk?

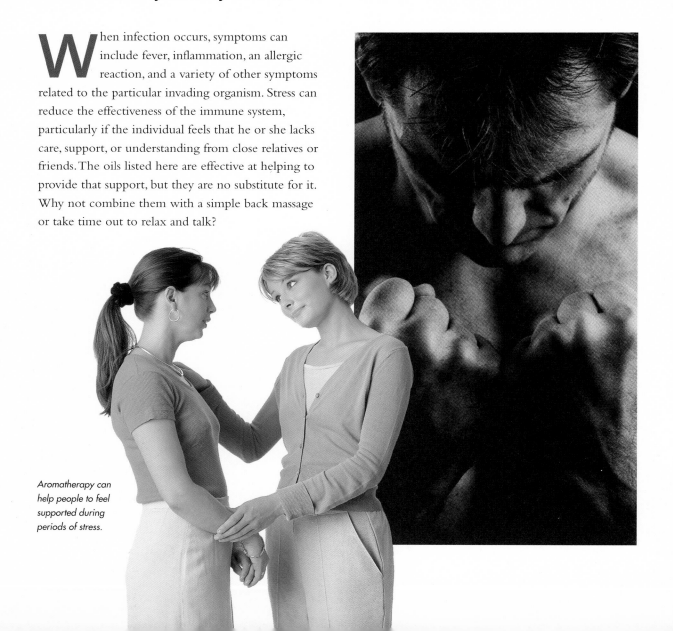

Aromatherapy can help people to feel supported during periods of stress.

IMMUNE SYSTEM

The immune system detects and fights foreign bodies, including unfriendly bacteria and invading organisms, and helps the body to resist infection and fend off disease. It uses a type of white blood cell, or lymphocyte, to produce antibodies.

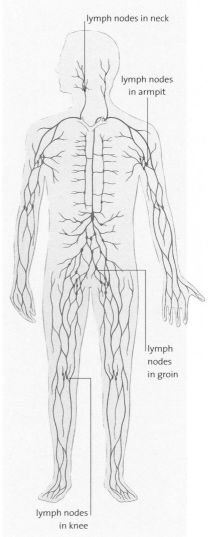

lymph nodes in neck

lymph nodes in armpit

lymph nodes in groin

lymph nodes in knee

DATA FILE

CONDITION	USEFUL ESSENTIAL OILS
Candidiasis or thrush	German camomile, lavender, lemon, lemongrass, manuka, may chang, niaouli, palmarosa, peppermint, tea tree, and yarrow
Chronic fatigue/glandular fever	Benzoin, black pepper, citriadora, eucalyptus, lemon, lemongrass, may chang, melissa, myrtle, ravensara, rose, tea tree, and yarrow
Immune-system deficiency—when the body can no longer fight infections or disease effectively, or you are continually getting colds or feeling run down	Bergamot, cardamom, grapefruit, lavender, lemon, lemongrass, manuka, may chang, melissa, pine, rose, rosewood, Roman camomile, tea tree, and ylang ylang
Cancer/tumors—these essential oils are particularly good at supporting people undergoing treatment. They are not a replacement for conventional treatment, but can help to alleviate some of the unpleasant side-effects	Bergamot, frankincense, lemon, lemongrass, melissa, niaouli, peppermint, and rose
Allergies and hypersensitivity	German camomile, lavender, lemon, rose, and yarrow

A wide range of essential oils, such as grapefruit, lavender, lemongrass, or bergamot, can help to soothe a sore throat and fatigue caused by glandular fever.

May chang Litsea cubeba

May chang is related to rosewood. Its light, lemony fragrance is similar to melissa and to lemongrass, and it does offer some of the same properties. May chang is wonderfully uplifting for people who are faced with a long recovery period from illness.

May chang helps ease postnatal depression and encourages milk production in breastfeeding mothers.

The wonderfully uplifting properties of may chang are ideal for people recovering from illness.

DATA FILE

GROWN IN: China

IN A BLEND: 3 drops in 4 teaspoons /20 ml of carrier oil (see pages 92–3)

FOR THE BODY: may chang is an effective antifungal oil, particularly for candida and vaginal and oral thrush. May chang is also used to support the immune system and is particularly effective for people recovering from chronic fatigue, cancer treatment, or frequent and long-term bouts of respiratory infections. In women, may chang can help ease painful periods and encourage milk production. It is also closely linked to the muscular system, and eases aches and pains, colitis, and diarrhea. May chang can also clear acne and balance the sebum production in oily skin.

FOR THE MIND: may chang is a mild stimulant, and its uplifting effects can help to ease postnatal depression, apathy, depression, lethargy and anxiety.

BLENDS WELL WITH: palmarosa, manuka, lavender, tea tree, eucalyptus, rosemary, geranium, jasmine, nutmeg, ginger, cedarwood, sandalwood, rosewood, frankincense, peppermint, vetiver, neroli, and thyme.

SAFETY NOTE
there is a mild risk of an allergic reaction; reduce the dose for people with sensitive skin.

Cedarwood Cedrus atlantica

Since it was first discovered, cedarwood has been used to build temples and items of spiritual significance. Biblical references to it abound, as do references to cedars in other world religions, including the tree's ability to uplift and provide strength in times of crisis. On a more mundane level, its fragrant wood is still used to store clothes and repel insects.

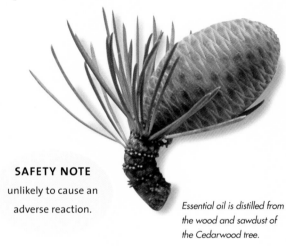

SAFETY NOTE
unlikely to cause an adverse reaction.

Essential oil is distilled from the wood and sawdust of the Cedarwood tree.

Cedarwood has long been associated with spirituality, and can be found in many different temples around the world.

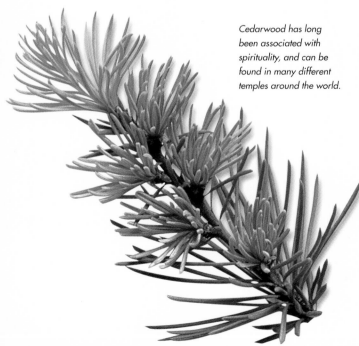

DATA FILE

GROWN IN: Morocco, Algeria

IN A BLEND: 2 drops in 4 teaspoons/20 ml of carrier oil (see pages 92–3)

FOR THE BODY: cedarwood is a strong antiseptic and astringent oil, and is particularly effective at clearing skin conditions such as acne, eczema, and psoriasis, as well as balancing oily and dry skin, clearing dandruff, and easing the itching associated with dermatitis or mosquito bites. Its antiseptic properties are also useful for clearing the symptoms associated with urinary tract infections, cystitis, and gonorrhea. This woody oil is also closely linked with the respiratory tract and is a gentle expectorant. It helps to clear bronchitis and catarrh, and eases both dry and hacking coughs, as well as reducing the severity of asthma attacks.

FOR THE MIND: cedarwood is a gentle sedative, easing anxiety and nervous tension.

BLENDS WELL WITH: sandalwood, frankincense, lavender, lemon, vetiver, rosewood, palmarosa, German camomile, yarrow, Roman camomile, benzoin, pine, niaouli, neroli, rose, geranium, jasmine, orange, bergamot, lemon, grapefruit, and coriander.

Cedarwood is a gentle, yet highly effective expectorant, which can aid those who suffer from asthma and ease attacks.

Seville bitter orange flowers, which bloom in Spain, France, Italy, and North Africa, are the source of neroli essential oil.

Neroli

Citrus aurantium var. vulgaris

Neroli has long been associated with its ability to alleviate fears, mistrust, and anxiety. Its presence in Victorian bridal headdresses helped many a nervous or unwilling girl to the altar. It is a very effective essential oil for fear and shock: try inhaling a drop on a tissue when faced with a crisis and there is no time for a massage.

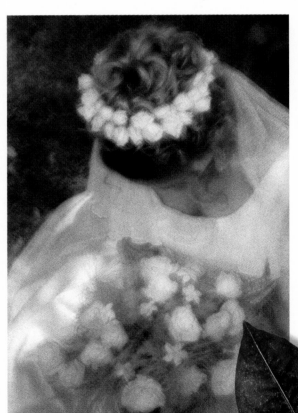

The soothing qualities of neroli are very effective for alleviating fears, and helped many young Victorian brides to overcome wedding nerves.

DATA FILE

GROWN IN: Tunisia, France

IN A BLEND: 3 drops in 4 teaspoons/20 ml of carrier oil (see pages 92–3)

FOR THE BODY: neroli is closely associated with the skin. It eases stretch marks, clears broken veins, and reduces the fine lines associated with aging skin. It is also a mild antispasmodic and helps to quieten heart palpitations, as well as easing nervous diarrhea and indigestion. It is also very helpful during labor.

FOR THE MIND: neroli is one of the essential oils frequently used to combat the signs of stress, especially where stress has produced physical problems. This uplifting oil is particularly effective at easing exhaustion, anxiety, panic, hysteria, shock, fear, depression, stress-related digestive upsets, insomnia, impatience, moodiness, and grief.

BLENDS WELL WITH: sandalwood, cedarwood, frankincense, vetiver, patchouli, coriander, nutmeg, clary sage, rose, cypress, ylang ylang, peppermint, ginger, jasmine, rosewood, melissa, and fennel.

SAFETY NOTE
unlikely to cause any
adverse reactions.

Bergamot Citrus bergamia var. communis

Bergamot is the flavoring behind Earl Grey tea and is one of the main ingredients of eau de Cologne. Its fresh, airy fragrance lifts the spirits immediately. It has been in use as an antiseptic and fever remedy since the 16th century, and is still a favorite with aromatherapists today.

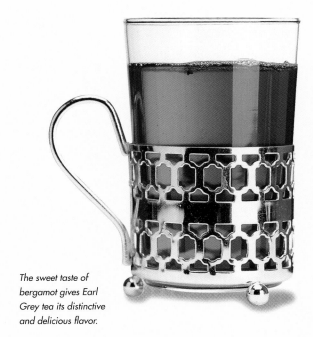

The sweet taste of bergamot gives Earl Grey tea its distinctive and delicious flavor.

SAFETY NOTE
For 12 hours after using at this concentration, avoid using sunbeds and UV light, or sitting in the sun. Bergamot can sensitize the skin to sunlight and may increase the risk of skin cancer.

DATA FILE

GROWN IN: Italy, France, Sicily

IN A BLEND: up to 4 drops in 4 teaspoons /20 ml of carrier oil (see pages 92–3)

FOR THE BODY: bergamot is an effective antiseptic and cell-rejuvenating oil. It is particularly effective at clearing acne, boils, eczema, dermatitis, and psoriasis and helps to heal varicose ulcers and cold sores. It also eases nervous indigestion, gastric reflux, belching, flatulence, and irritable bowel syndrome. Bergamot can also be used to support the immune system—especially for conditions such as pharyngitis, urogenital infections, chronic fatigue, and the side effects of cancer treatment.

FOR THE MIND: bergamot is very uplifting. Use it for anxiety, depression, mood swings, insomnia, and nightmares.

BLENDS WELL WITH: lavender, cedarwood, yarrow, Roman camomile, German camomile, frankincense, patchouli, palmarosa, lemongrass, rosemary, peppermint, geranium, rose, neroli, sandalwood, melissa, clary sage, and marjoram.

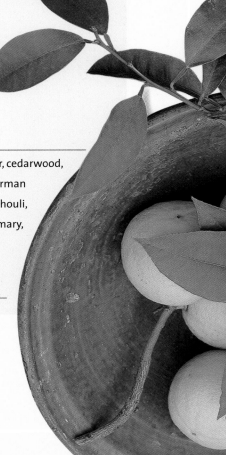

Bergamot essential oil is expressed from the peel of the fruit when it is nearly ripe. It has a fresh, sweet, uplifting smell.

Melissa Melissa officinalis

Otherwise known as lemon balm, melissa's sweet lemon fragrance has wafted through sun-drenched gardens for generations. It was first introduced to Europe by the Romans, and was used at that time for its gentle healing effects on conditions as wide-ranging as toothache, headaches and asthma.

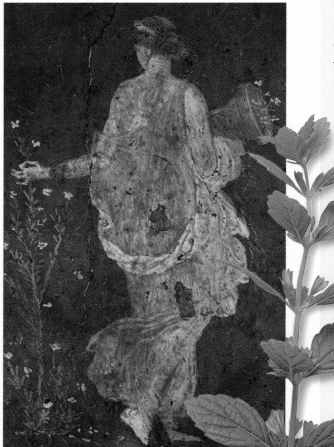

The lemon balm plant has a refreshing lemon scent and flavor, and has been used for centuries to help treat a wide range of ailments from toothache, headache, and fatigue, to the common cold and other viral infections.

DATA FILE

GROWN IN: Spain, France, North Africa

IN A BLEND: 2 drops in 4 teaspoons/20 ml of carrier oil (see pages 92–3)

FOR THE BODY: melissa is particularly useful for reducing the effects and aftereffects of viral infections such as cold sores, shingles, genital herpes, impetigo, influenza, chronic fatigue, and colds. It is also a useful antispasmodic, and can help to ease painful periods, heart palpitations, headaches, and migraines. It can also help to lower blood pressure.

FOR THE MIND: melissa eases panic, shock, and insomnia, helps improve faulty memories, helps ease the cravings associated with tranquilizer or alcohol addiction, encourages serenity and eases anxious depression and fear.

BLENDS WELL WITH: fennel, clary sage, sandalwood, palmarosa, patchouli, jasmine, vetiver, cedarwood, frankincense, juniper, marjoram, Roman camomile, geranium, rose, neroli, carrot seed, benzoin, bay, niaouli, tea tree, and lavender.

SAFETY NOTE
there is a minimal risk of allergic reaction. To be sure, do a patch test on sensitive, diseased, or damaged skin.

Petitgrain Citrus
aurantium var. amara

The fruit from the Seville bitter orange tree is used to make marmalade, and has little medicinal benefit when used in this way.

Petitgrain is extracted from the leaves and twigs of the Seville bitter orange tree. It is invaluable for clearing digestive difficulties as well as for uplifting the mind and relieving depression. It has been a common ingredient of many perfumes developed over the last two centuries.

Petitgrain is distilled from the leaves and twigs of the Seville bitter orange tree (the flowers are used to produce neroli oil—see page 44).

SAFETY NOTE
unlikely to cause an adverse reaction.

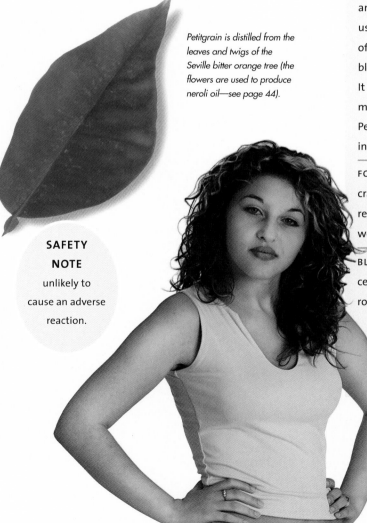

Petitgrain is excellent for relieving restlessness and agitation.

DATA FILE

GROWN IN: France, Paraguay, Italy, Egypt, Tunisia

IN A BLEND: 2 drops in 4 teaspoons/20 ml of carrier oil (see pages 92–3)

FOR THE BODY: petitgrain is an effective antiseptic and antispasmodic essential oil. It is particularly useful for supporting the digestive system in cases of gastric reflux, belching, hiccups, nausea, vomiting, bloating, discomfort, irritable bowel, and flatulence. It also helps to ease heart palpitations, general muscular aches and pains, catarrh, and bronchitis. Petitgrain can also ease excessive sweating and infected acne, and balance oily skin.

FOR THE MIND: petitgrain eases insomnia, addictive cravings, anxiety, panic attacks, nervousness, restlessness, nervous exhaustion, overthinking, worry, depression, agitation, and disillusionment

BLENDS WELL WITH: orange, neroli, sandalwood, cedarwood, bergamot, vetiver, palmarosa, rosewood, geranium, peppermint, ylang ylang, Roman camomile, yarrow, patchouli, lemon, fennel, jasmine, and benzoin.

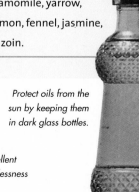

Protect oils from the sun by keeping them in dark glass bottles.

Aromatherapy **massage** for the **back**

When you are giving a person a massage, look after your own back by maintaining good posture. If you do not have access to a massage couch, then ask the person to lie on towels on the floor for the treatment, while you kneel beside him or her. If working on the floor sounds too painful, ask the person to straddle a chair and stand behind to carry out the treatment.

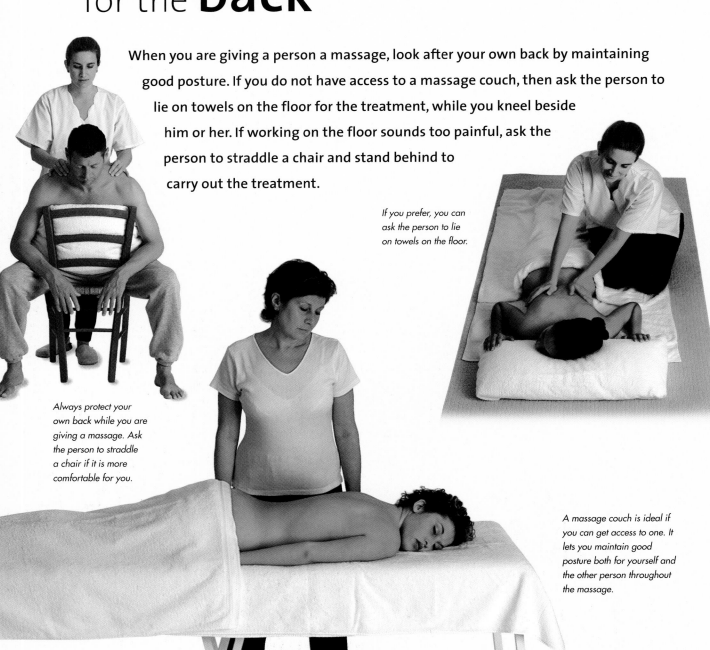

If you prefer, you can ask the person to lie on towels on the floor.

Always protect your own back while you are giving a massage. Ask the person to straddle a chair if it is more comfortable for you.

A massage couch is ideal if you can get access to one. It lets you maintain good posture both for yourself and the other person throughout the massage.

BACK MASSAGE

1 Standing to the person's left, gradually lower your hands to the person's back, one hand at the base of the skull, and the other over the sacrum (lower back). Hold for a count of 20, or until the skin under your hands starts to get hot and you feel the person beginning to relax.

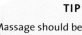

TIP
Massage should be enjoyable and soothing so, from time to time, check with the person you are massaging that there is no discomfort.

2 Apply the oil in smooth, flowing strokes, working up the body from the waist to the shoulders. The pressure is always upwards—toward the heart. This movement is called effleurage. When you reach the shoulders, glide your hands gently down the sides of the body and repeat the movement three times. You can then do the same upward movement in smaller areas—over the waist (three times), then mid-back, followed by shoulders. Effleurage helps to relax the person and warm up the area that you are massaging. It also gives you a chance to work out where the person is most tense.

Use smooth, flowing strokes. Work the oil up the back from the waist to the shoulders.

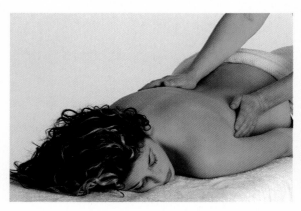

When you reach the shoulders, let your hands slide down the sides of the body toward the lower back.

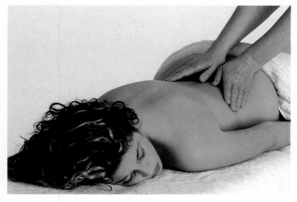

Bring your hands together at the lower back, before moving them up the back toward the shoulders again.

3 Kneading—for this movement, you pick up the flesh in one hand before passing it to the other in a push-pull or side-to-side movement. This is exactly like kneading bread. Start with the flesh at the hip and work up the body to the shoulders on both sides of the body. Spend some time over the shoulders —this is where a lot of people store their stress. The muscles get extremely tight here, especially if the person has spent all day hunched over a computer or dealing with demanding toddlers.

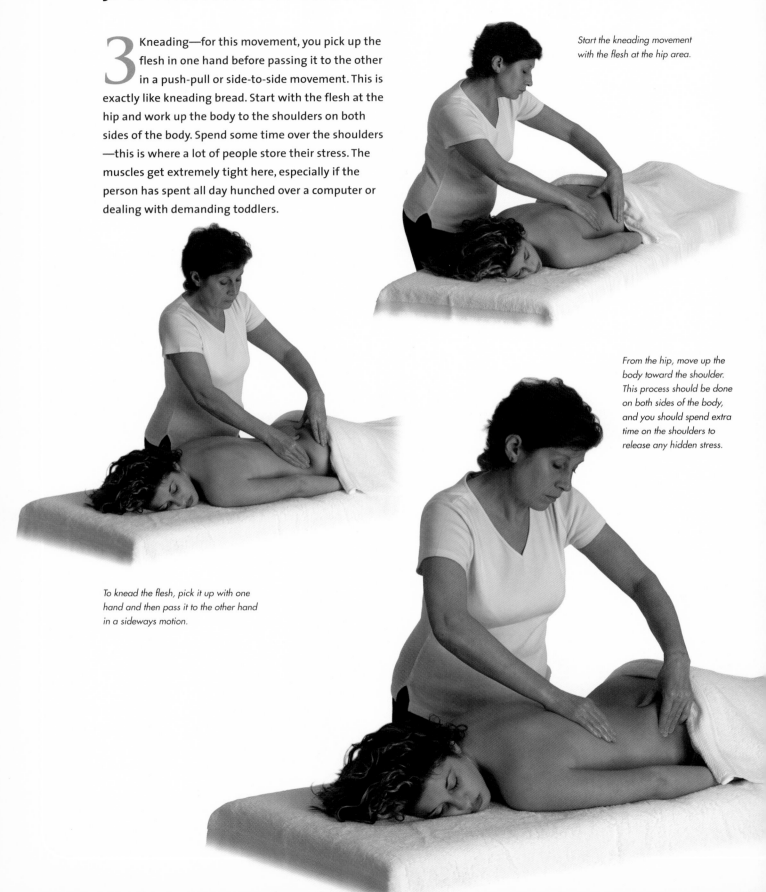

Start the kneading movement with the flesh at the hip area.

From the hip, move up the body toward the shoulder. This process should be done on both sides of the body, and you should spend extra time on the shoulders to release any hidden stress.

To knead the flesh, pick it up with one hand and then pass it to the other hand in a sideways motion.

4 Petrissage —this is a small, circular, grinding movement that you make with your thumbs, pushing tight muscle against the underlying bone. Make sure you have warmed up the area first with lots of effleurage and kneading. Keep the petrissage movements small, slow, and deep. Each circle you make is about the size of a quarter. Work along the erector spinae—the group of muscles that stand out on either side of the spine like two long chords—and around both shoulder blades. Repeat the petrissage as often as you like—and at least three times over each area.

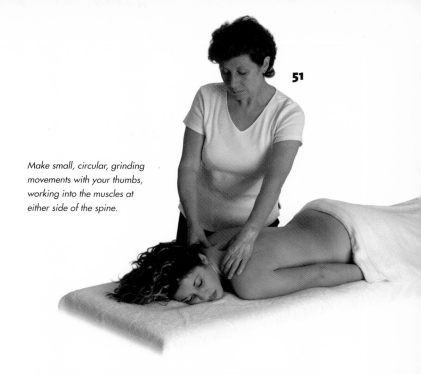

Make small, circular, grinding movements with your thumbs, working into the muscles at either side of the spine.

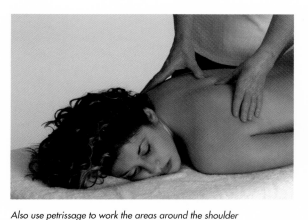

Also use petrissage to work the areas around the shoulder blades. People tend to store a lot of tension in these areas.

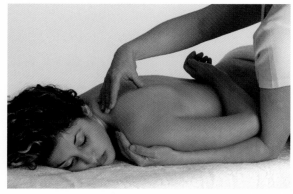

Knead the upper arm, then bring the lower arm up and rotate the upper arm from the shoulder joint.

5 Repeat kneading from step 3, this time incorporating kneading to the upper arm, and rotate the arm from the shoulder joint. This movement helps to loosen up tight shoulders and reminds the person to hold the shoulders back (and stand up straight).

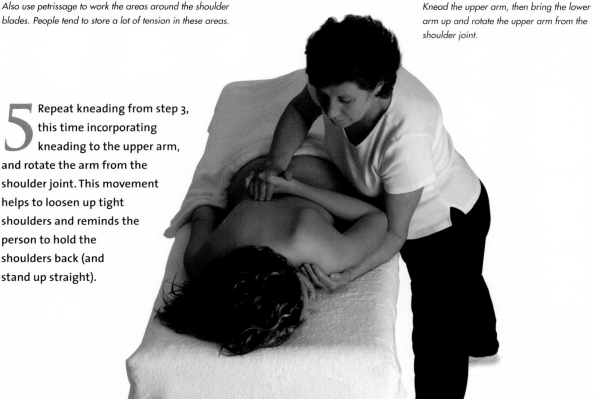

6 Knuckling—if you find that petrissage is painful to carry out, or the person you are massaging has extremely tight shoulders or is very muscle-bound, use your knuckles instead. This movement uses the knuckles of the first joint of your fingers. Place your knuckles on your friend's back, then rotate your hands from the wrists (as if they were eggbeaters). This movement is very effective at increasing blood circulation to the area. Try it over the upper back and into the upper shoulders.

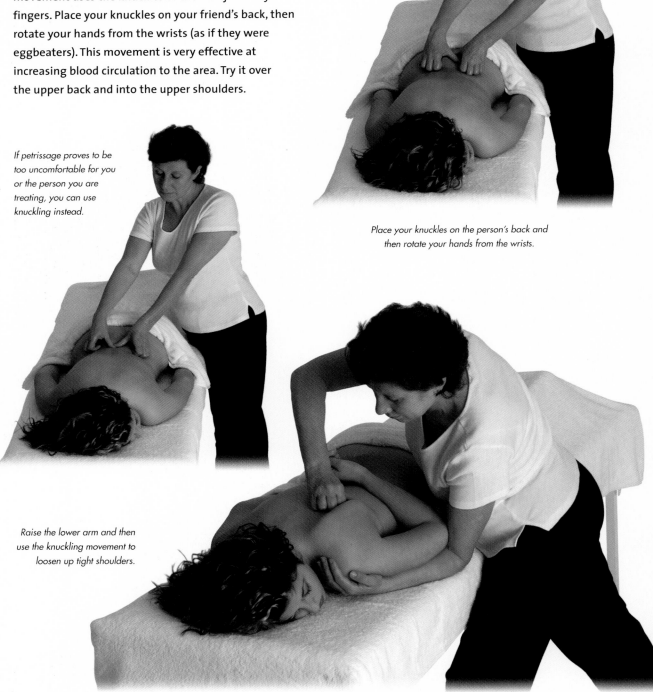

If petrissage proves to be too uncomfortable for you or the person you are treating, you can use knuckling instead.

Place your knuckles on the person's back and then rotate your hands from the wrists.

Raise the lower arm and then use the knuckling movement to loosen up tight shoulders.

7 Forearm sweep—place your forearm alongside the spine with your elbow just above the buttocks. Clasp the working hand with your other hand for support. Lean into the movement and slide your forearm all the way up the back, and over the shoulder. Lift your arm off gently, and repeat twice for each side of the spine.

8 Repeat effleurage from step 2, although this time the emphasis of movement is outward (from the spine to the sides of the body).

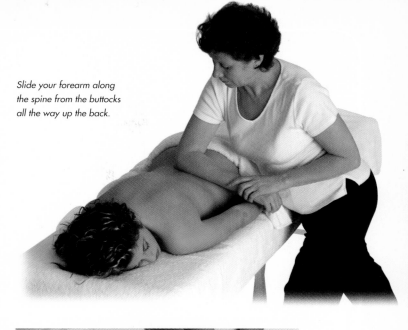

Slide your forearm along the spine from the buttocks all the way up the back.

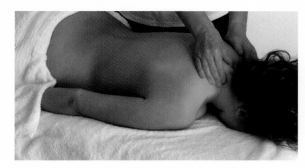

Move your hands in smooth, flowing strokes outward from the spine to the sides of the body, then move them to the base of the skull. Knead the neck and do some gentle petrissage.

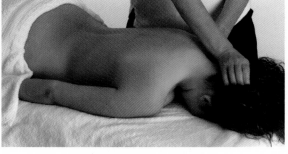

Give the neck a slight stretch by holding the base of the skull and putting some gentle pressure upward toward the skull.

9 Use one hand to knead the neck, followed by gentle petrissage, followed by a hold at the base of the skull and a slight pressure upward toward the skull. This gives the neck a gentle stretch.

10 Repeat the petrissage movements to either side of the spine.

11 Repeat effleurage from step 2 to finish the massage. Cover the person with a towel.

TIP

If the person you are treating has any history of back pain or neck injury, you should consult a qualified medical practitioner first.

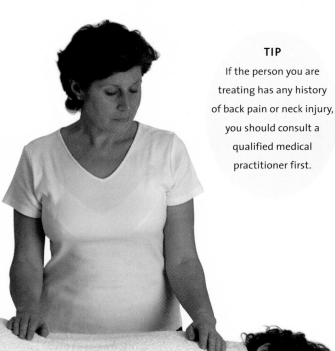

The **feel-good** factor: aromatherapy and the **emotions**

So many of the essential oils distilled and used today are chosen for their ability to evoke pleasant memories in addition to their effects on your physical body. Try palmarosa to cool feelings of frustration; benzoin or sandalwood to ease tension or poor communication; frankincense to instill calm or promote meditation; neroli for shock or rose for grief.

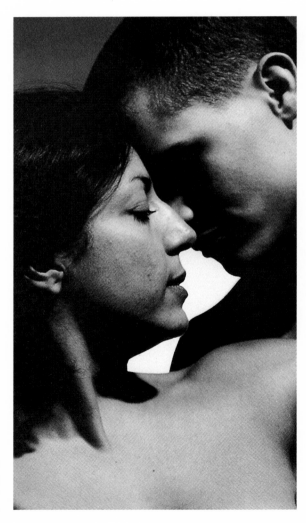

Stress can leave the individual feeling emotionally wrought. Whether the symptoms manifest themselves as insomnia, restlessness, fear, or depression, essential oils will help to balance your outlook on life, improve the quality of your sleep, and allay your fears. However, even lavender, that well-known sedative, can sometimes fail to change unsettled sleeping patterns. If this happens, you can try blending it with something more uplifting like geranium, or substitute it for a stronger sedative such as Roman camomile.

If you, or someone you love, are experiencing more severe difficulties, and perhaps have even developed bad eating patterns, it is important to look at the underlying causes of the condition. In such a case, turn to a qualified doctor, or a trained counselor or psychotherapist; this can make an enormous difference between "soldiering on" ineffectively and returning to good health.

Lavender is a very effective sedative and can help to regulate unsettled sleeping patterns.

Essential oils such as sandalwood and ylang ylang can help restore lost sex drive.

DATA FILE

CONDITION	USEFUL ESSENTIAL OILS
Anxiety/ insomnia	Camomile maroc, German camomile, Clary sage, cypress, lavender, marjoram, melissa, neroli, Roman camomile, rosewood, valerian, vetiver, and yarrow
Depression	Bergamot, cedarwood, clary sage, frankincense, geranium, grapefruit, jasmine, lemongrass, may chang, melissa, neroli, nutmeg, orange, rose, Roman camomile, and ylang ylang
Panic attacks	Lavender, marjoram, melissa, neroli, and valerian
Lack of appetite/ irregular eating patterns	Black pepper, frankincense, geranium, ginger, grapefruit, jasmine, juniper, neroli, orange, patchouli, peppermint, rose, rosemary, vetiver, or ylang ylang
Recovery from addictions – reducing cravings associated with addictions to substances such as alcohol, tranquilizers, caffeine, and nicotine	Carrot seed, clary sage, fennel, frankincense, lavender, lemon, melissa, patchouli, rose, valerian, vetiver, yarrow, and ylang ylang
Loss of sex drive	Black pepper, cedarwood, clary sage, damiana, jasmine, patchouli, rose, sandalwood, vetiver, and ylang ylang

LEMON

Essential oils, such as ginger and grapefruit, can help people suffering from lack of appetite to establish normal eating patterns.

Cycles in life: aromatherapy and the **reproductive** system

The reproductive system is not essential for immediate survival, which is why so many women under stress note a change in their menstrual cycle. This is because processes that are not essential for survival come to a halt when the "fight or flight" response swings into action. The reproductive system does, however, play an important role in our lives and in many cases our identity and self-awareness is tied up in our reproductive ability. For women, it also provides a reminder that there is a cycle of sorts running through life.

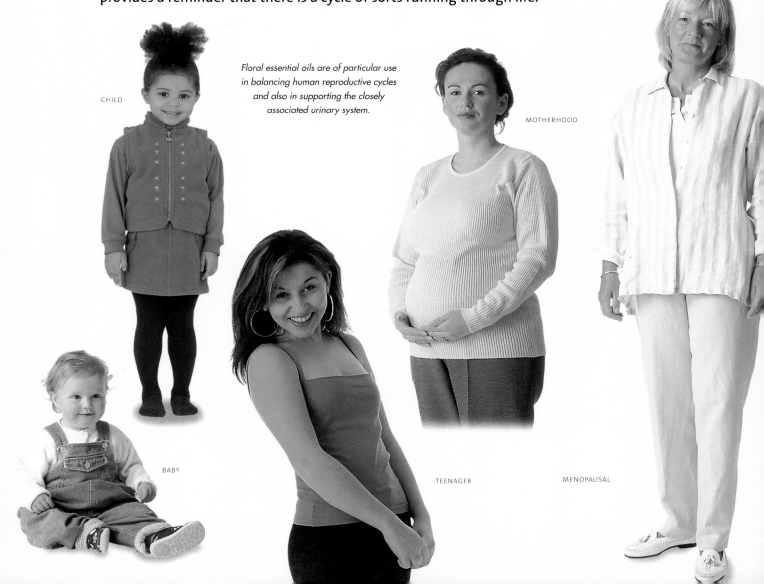

Floral essential oils are of particular use in balancing human reproductive cycles and also in supporting the closely associated urinary system.

CHILD

MOTHERHOOD

BABY

TEENAGER

MENOPAUSAL

DATA FILE

CONDITION	USEFUL ESSENTIAL OILS
Premenstrual tension (PMT)	Bergamot, clary sage, cypress, damiana, frankincense, geranium, grapefruit, melissa, neroli, Roman camomile, rose, and ylang ylang
Irregular menses/lack of periods	Clary sage, damiana, fennel, geranium, jasmine, juniper, peppermint, Roman camomile, rose, and ylang ylang
Painful periods	Clary sage, cypress, geranium, German camomile, lavender, marjoram, peppermint, Roman camomile, rose, and valerian
Heavy periods	Clary sage, cypress, frankincense, lavender, lemon, peppermint, and Roman camomile
Menopausal symptoms including night sweats, changing menstrual cycle, hot flushes, aching joints, changing quality of the skin, insomnia, and heart palpitations	Bergamot, clary sage, cypress, damiana, fennel, geranium, grapefruit, may chang, palmarosa, Roman camomile, rose, spikenard, valerian, and ylang ylang
Thrush	Lavender, lemon, manuka, niaouli, pine, and tea tree
Infertility in men and women	Black pepper, clary sage, fennel, geranium, jasmine, patchouli, rose, sandalwood, and vetiver
Endometriosis	Cypress, clary sage, frankincense, lavender, myrrh, and rose
Cystitis	Cypress, eucalyptus, geranium, juniper, lavender, lemon, manuka, rose, sandalwood, and tea tree
Incontinence	Cypress, damiana, rose, and yarrow
Prostatitis (inflamation of the prostate gland)	Jasmine, juniper, neroli, niaouli, pine, Roman camomile, tea tree, and yarrow

CAMOMILE LEAVES

OLD AGE

Geranium
Pelargonium graveolens

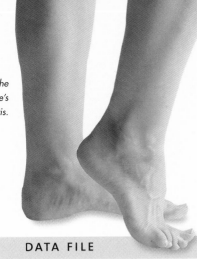

Geranium helps in the treatment of athlete's foot and dermatitis.

Geranium is a popular European garden plant, and its roselike fragrance means that it is one of the key ingredients used to adulterate its more expensive sister oil, rose. Thanks to its gentle, sweet, and uplifting aroma, geranium can be used for many of the same functions as those of a rose, and at a fraction of the price.

SAFETY NOTE
unlikely to cause an adverse reaction.

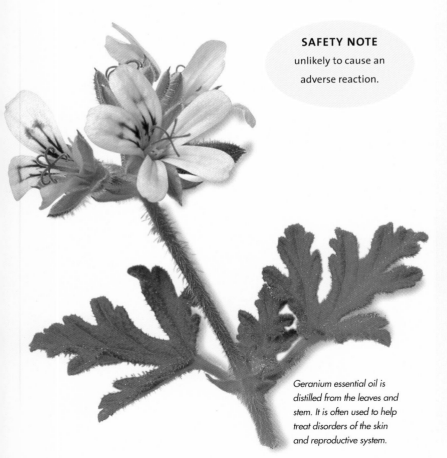

Geranium essential oil is distilled from the leaves and stem. It is often used to help treat disorders of the skin and reproductive system.

DATA FILE

GROWN IN: Réunion, North Africa, China, Egypt

IN A BLEND: 3 drops in 4 teaspoons/20 ml of carrier oil (see pages 92–3)

FOR THE BODY: geranium is most closely associated with the skin and the reproductive system. It is an effective essential oil and helps to ease the discomfort associated with dermatitis, dry/oily skin, eczema, cold sores, shingles, ringworm, hemorrhoids, psoriasis, athlete's foot, impetigo, boils, painful periods, fibroids, fluid retention, hormonal imbalances, swollen breasts, menstrual irregularity, premenstrual tension, pregnancy, cystitis and night sweats. It can improve the appearance of stretch marks and varicose veins and provides some support for the digestive system, easing colitis, diarrhea, peptic ulcers, acid indigestion, gastroenteritis and gallstones.

FOR THE MIND: geranium is commonly used to ease anxiety, depression, postnatal depression, emotional and nervous exhaustion, mood swings, overwork, and insomnia.

BLENDS WELL WITH: cedarwood, rosewood, frankincense, lemon, marjoram, lemongrass, petitgrain, patchouli, vetiver, sandalwood, grapefruit, rosemary, peppermint, melissa, fennel, cypress, myrrh, lavender, damiana, tea tree, and manuka.

Damiana Turnera diffusa

Damiana is frequently used in Central and South America as an ingredient in relaxing herbal teas designed to aid digestion and heal the mind. Its gentle, apple-like aroma makes it a wonderful, comforting essential oil to use. Try it with Roman camomile, rose, or bergamot to evoke the smell of warm sunny days in a garden.

SAFETY NOTE

unlikely to cause an adverse reaction.

Dried damiana is often used in herbal teas. Damiana is a small shrub that grows in South America.

Damiana tea is uplifting and helps to counter physical weakness and nervous exhaustion.

DATA FILE

GROWN IN: Mexico, Brazil and Central America

IN A BLEND: 2 drops in 4 teaspoons/20 ml of carrier oil (see pages 92–3)

FOR THE BODY: damiana is particularly effective for supporting the digestive, reproductive, and endocrine systems. Use it for constipation, irritable bowel, irregular or painful periods, premenstrual tension, lack of appetite, chronic fatigue, cystitis, or hormone imbalances.

FOR THE MIND: damiana is an uplifting oil. Use it for chronic exhaustion, loss of sexual drive, disturbed eating patterns, depression, or anxiety.

BLENDS WELL WITH: rose, neroli, geranium, Roman camomile, yarrow, vetiver, juniper, peppermint, bergamot, orange, black pepper, fennel, valerian, and sandalwood.

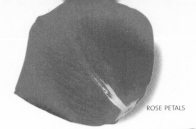

ROSE PETALS

Rose Rosa damascena

'A rose by any other name would not smell as sweet'—humanity's long-standing love-affair with roses began long before Shakespeare placed Juliet on her balcony. Ancient Greeks dedicated the blossoms to Aphrodite, the goddess of love and beauty—which was a highly appropriate choice given the essential oil's strong aphrodisiac qualities and its link to fertility and the reproductive system.

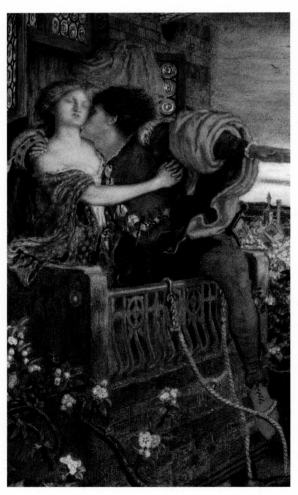

Flowers and fragrances make many appearances in Shakespeare's plays, and the rose is prominent in Romeo and Juliet.

DATA FILE

GROWN IN: Bulgaria, Turkey, France

IN A BLEND: 1 drop in 4 teaspoons/20 ml of carrier oil (see pages 92–3)

FOR THE BODY: rose is closely linked to the reproductive system, skin, and liver. Use it to ease the symptoms of cold sores, shingles, pruritis, inflamed skin, irregular or painful menstruation, to balance hormones during menopause, to prepare the uterus for labor during the last three months of pregnancy, for endometriosis, fibroids, cirrhosis, insufficient bile production, and during recovery from addiction to substances such as alcohol and nicotine. Rose also helps ease stress-related immune-system conditions.

FOR THE MIND: rose is an effective aphrodisiac. It also helps deal with forgotten emotional wounds, repressed anger, envy, resentment, impatience, confusion, depression, loss of sexual drive, frustration, jealousy, and nervous exhaustion.

BLENDS WELL WITH: frankincense, neroli, orange, sandalwood, vetiver, patchouli, clary sage, fennel, nutmeg, cedarwood, Roman camomile, damiana, lemon, grapefruit, orange, petitgrain, peppermint, ginger, and coriander.

SAFETY NOTE
unlikely to cause an
adverse reaction.

Sandalwood Santalum album

The heavenly scent of sandalwood is highly valued as a perfume and incense ingredient. The wood is still used throughout South-east Asia to create religious icons and small pieces of furniture. It has sensual and aphrodisiac qualities that soothe the nervous system. Aromatherapists prize it for its beneficial effect on conditions associated with the skin and the lungs.

DATA FILE

GROWN IN: India

IN A BLEND: 3 drops in 4 teaspoons/20 ml of carrier oil (see pages 92–3)

FOR THE BODY: sandalwood helps to clear acne and balance oily or dry skin. It also helps to ease dermatitis, eczema, psoriasis, chronic bronchitis, laryngitis, catarrh, mucous, coughs, and sore throats and to clear varicose veins and hemorrhoids. It is also extremely useful in treating cystitis.

FOR THE MIND: use sandalwood to soothe fear, paranoia, lack of confidence or loss of sexual drive, restlessness, and insomnia.

BLENDS WELL WITH: vetiver, cedarwood, bergamot, grapefruit, orange, mandarin, benzoin, clove, frankincense, patchouli, geranium, rose, neroli, cypress, myrrh, pine, manuka, and lavender.

SAFETY NOTE
unlikely to cause an
adverse reaction.

Sandalwood incense balances the mind, body, and spirit.

The essential oil is extracted from the inner wood of the tree, and also from the roots. Sandalwood soothes fear and is a decongestant.

Palmarosa
Cymbopogon martini var. martini

Palmarosa fragrance is very popular and nowadays can often be found in many cosmetics and perfumes.

Palmarosa was used in the 18th century to adulterate rose. Its light, floral, and grassy aroma is still a popular fragrance found in soaps, cosmetics, and perfumes. Palmarosa is an extremely effective essential oil in the treatment of skin and it also helps to cool anger, jealousy, and insecurity.

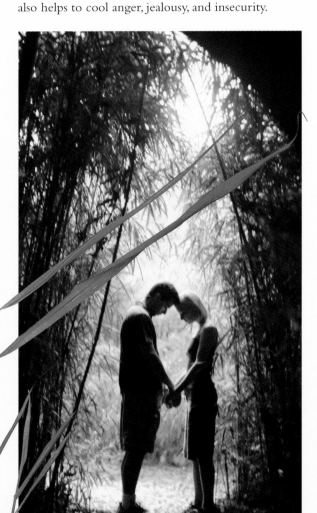

LEFT *Palmarosa is soothing and helps to ease feelings of anger, jealousy, or insecurity.*

FAR LEFT *Palmarosa is a grass and grows in India, Indonesia, Africa, and South America. The whole plant is used for extracting the aromatic essential oil.*

DATA FILE

GROWN IN: Brazil, India, Madagascar

IN A BLEND: 3 drops in 4 teaspoons/20 ml of carrier oil (see pages 92–3)

FOR THE BODY: palmarosa is closely linked to the skin and digestive and reproductive systems. Use it for acne, oily skin, infected or inflamed skin, dry skin, eczema, psoriasis, colitis, and gastroenteritis. It is also useful for treating reproductive-system disorders such as pelvic inflammatory conditions, thrush, and cystitis.

FOR THE MIND: eases anger, jealousy, rage, and mood swings.

BLENDS WELL WITH: lemon, patchouli, vetiver, lemongrass, frankincense, neroli, jasmine, rose, cedarwood, and orange

SAFETY NOTE
unlikely to cause an adverse reaction.

Jasmine Jasminum officinale

Jasmine is an ingredient in many popular perfumes. Its link with fertility, sensuality, and love dates back to its appearance in Hindu artwork featuring Kama, the god of love, whose arrows were tipped with jasmine blossoms. Their musky scent is guaranteed to lift anxiety and depression and pierce the heart of any lover.

SAFETY NOTE
slight risk of allergic skin reaction. Use with care on sensitive skin or where the skin is compromised in some way.

Jasmine has strong aprhodisiac qualities and has been linked with love and sensuality for centuries.

DATA FILE

GROWN IN: North Africa, France, China, India

IN A BLEND: 2 drops in 4 teaspoons/20 ml of carrier oil (see pages 92–3)

FOR THE BODY: jasmine is particularly supportive during pregnancy and childbirth. Use it in the last three months of pregnancy only, for engorged breasts and for insufficient milk supply. It can also be used for irregular or painful periods, and dry and greasy skin. In men, it is particularly useful for easing the symptoms of prostatitis.

FOR THE MIND: jasmine is a strong aphrodisiac, and is useful for apathy, depression, emotional coldness, loss of sexual drive, lack of confidence, insomnia, and nervous exhaustion.

BLENDS WELL WITH: frankincense, patchouli, melissa, vetiver, sandalwood, palmarosa, lemongrass, ginger, fennel, bergamot, black pepper, coriander, rosewood, grapefruit, and lemon.

Jasmine grows in France, North Africa, and the Far East. Only the flowers are used for the oil.

Self-massage for **neck** and **shoulder** pain

You can now buy a number of products that feel like bean bags and contain wheat or rice loaded with essential oils. They are heated in a microwave oven for a couple of minutes and then placed on sore points to soothe aching muscles. The essential oils help to reduce stress as well.

Place a warmed aromatherapy cushion on sore muscles.

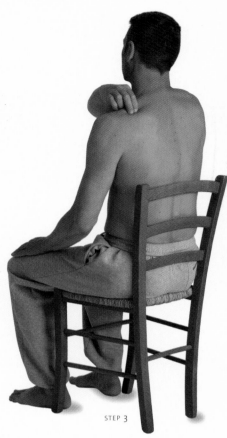

STEP 3

If a massage therapist is unavailable, you can still give yourself a very effective massage to relieve pain in your neck and shoulders and reduce discomfort in your chest.

1 Grasp and hold as large a handful of muscle as you can manage. Hold for 10 seconds, then release.

2 Knead into the area (see page 50), working firmly to loosen up the tight muscles.

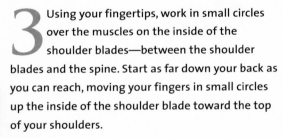

STEP 2

3 Using your fingertips, work in small circles over the muscles on the inside of the shoulder blades—between the shoulder blades and the spine. Start as far down your back as you can reach, moving your fingers in small circles up the inside of the shoulder blade toward the top of your shoulders.

TIP

If you have tender or swollen breasts as a result of pregnancy, breastfeeding, mastitis, painful periods, or premenstrual tension, you can incorporate massage to the breasts in this treatment. Keep the movement to a simple, smooth effleurage stroke working from the sternum—breastbone—out to the armpits. Alternate your movements, with one stroke to the underside of the breast followed by one stroke to the upper side of the breast, always finishing at the armpit. This helps to move any swelling or lymphatic congestion into the lymph nodes in this area. Try lavender, Roman camomile, cypress, or geranium for best results.

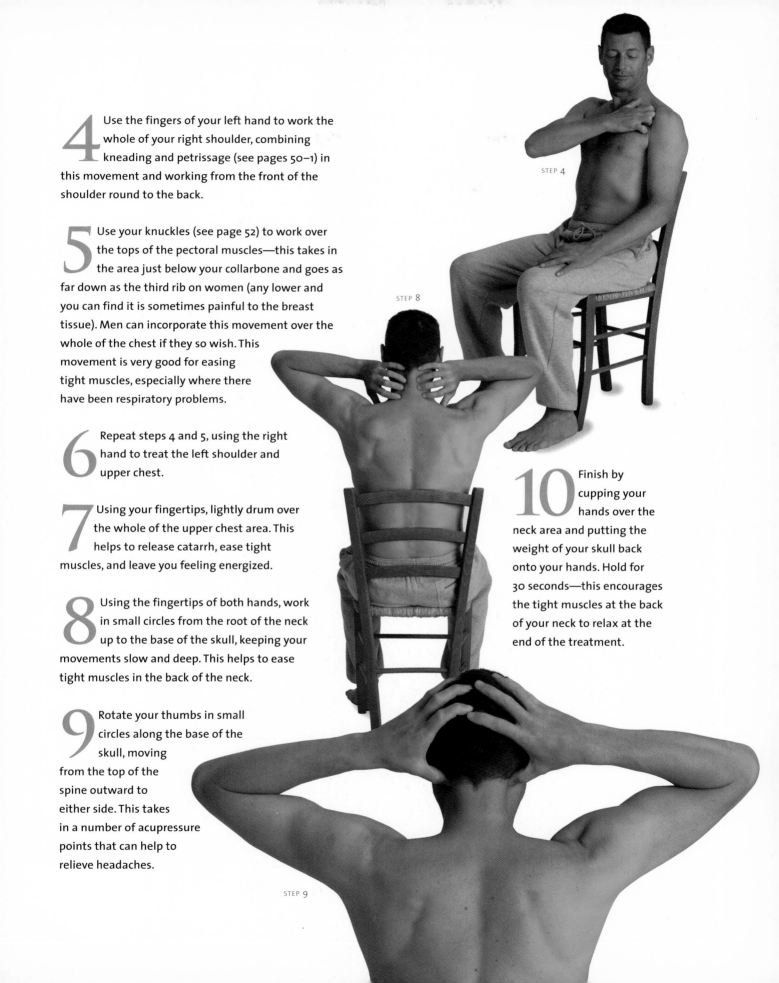

4 Use the fingers of your left hand to work the whole of your right shoulder, combining kneading and petrissage (see pages 50–1) in this movement and working from the front of the shoulder round to the back.

5 Use your knuckles (see page 52) to work over the tops of the pectoral muscles—this takes in the area just below your collarbone and goes as far down as the third rib on women (any lower and you can find it is sometimes painful to the breast tissue). Men can incorporate this movement over the whole of the chest if they so wish. This movement is very good for easing tight muscles, especially where there have been respiratory problems.

6 Repeat steps 4 and 5, using the right hand to treat the left shoulder and upper chest.

7 Using your fingertips, lightly drum over the whole of the upper chest area. This helps to release catarrh, ease tight muscles, and leave you feeling energized.

8 Using the fingertips of both hands, work in small circles from the root of the neck up to the base of the skull, keeping your movements slow and deep. This helps to ease tight muscles in the back of the neck.

9 Rotate your thumbs in small circles along the base of the skull, moving from the top of the spine outward to either side. This takes in a number of acupressure points that can help to relieve headaches.

10 Finish by cupping your hands over the neck area and putting the weight of your skull back onto your hands. Hold for 30 seconds—this encourages the tight muscles at the back of your neck to relax at the end of the treatment.

STEP 4

STEP 8

STEP 9

Catch your breath:
the **respiratory** system

The respiratory system is one of the first places where many of us note the effects of stress on our bodies. You might become prone to coughs and colds, or you could develop asthma following a chest infection or have difficulty breathing when you are under stress. While the immune system is definitely involved in some of these conditions, such as asthma, we still experience discomfort in the lungs and chest and special measures need to be taken.

One of the things that happens to a lot of people under stress is that they start to breathe more shallowly, using only the top third of their lungs. You see this particularly when someone is asthmatic. Learning to breathe more deeply, from your diaphragm (situated at the base of your ribs, just above your stomach), so that the whole of your lungs are inflated with each inhalation, can make a huge difference, not only to the health of your lungs but also to your state of mind. Give yourself, literally, time to catch your breath. Many essential oils are particularly effective here at encouraging pain-free breathing, clearing catarrh, and helping you to relax and breathe more deeply. If you have access to an electric vaporizer, try steaming some of these oils—frankincense, cedarwood, marjoram or benzoin—next to your bed at night to encourage restful sleep without coughing. (Do not leave candles or naked flames burning unattended.)

Many essential oils can encourage pain-free breathing.

Try steaming oils in a vaporizer.

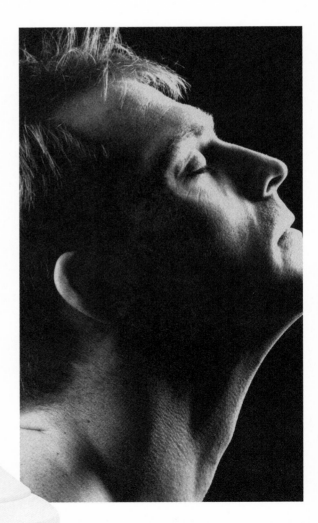

DATA FILE

CONDITION	USEFUL ESSENTIAL OILS
Asthma	Eucalyptus, frankincense, lavender, lemon, niaouli, pine, Roman camomile, rose otto, and sandalwood
Bronchitis	Black pepper, clove, cypress, eucalyptus, frankincense, ginger, juniper, lemon, marjoram, myrrh, niaouli, pine, rose otto, sandalwood, tea tree, and thyme
Catarrh	Benzoin, black pepper, cedarwood, lemon, marjoram, niaouli, peppermint, and rosemary
Coughs/colds	Black pepper, cedarwood, cypress, eucalyptus, geranium, juniper, lavender, lemon, marjoram, peppermint, pine, tea tree, and thyme
Earache	Basil, Roman camomile, lavender, and rosemary
Infections	Frankincense, lemon, niaouli, petitgrain, pine, rosewood, and thyme
Influenza	Eucalyptus, clove, myrrh, niaouli, peppermint, pine, rosemary, thyme, basil, and black pepper
Laryngitis	Black pepper, cypress, eucalyptus, lemon, myrrh, niaouli, peppermint, and sandalwood
Sinusitis	Basil, clove, eucalyptus, marjoram, niaouli, peppermint, pine, rosemary, tea tree, and thyme

LAVENDER

BASIL LEAVES

You can ease mild cases of earache by putting a few drops of essential oil onto a piece of absorbent cotton and holding it carefully against the outer ear. Try basil, Roman camomile, lavender, or rosemary.

DRIED ROMAN CAMOMILE

Benzoin Styrax benzoin

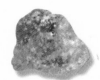

Benzoin has been used for generations as a remedy for chapped skin and various respiratory problems, and is one of the key ingredients in Friar's Balsam. This 14th-century remedy is still in use today—it is employed in some hospitals to help heal wounds following dermatological operations and around catheters to keep infection at bay.

SAFETY NOTE
unlikely to cause an adverse reaction.

Benzoin gum comes from a shrubby tree that grows in tropical rainforests in South-East Asia.

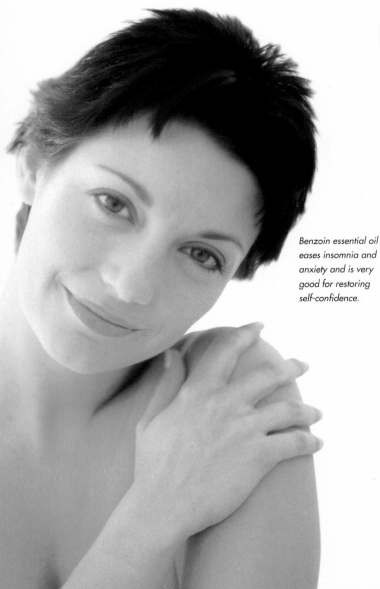

Benzoin essential oil eases insomnia and anxiety and is very good for restoring self-confidence.

DATA FILE

GROWN IN: Malaysia, Java, Sumatra, Thailand, China

IN A BLEND: 2 drops in 20 ml/4 teaspoons carrier oil (see pages 92–3)

FOR THE BODY: benzoin is closely associated with the respiratory system and the skin, and is extremely effective at easing the symptoms of bronchitis, catarrh, coughs, asthma, wheezing, laryngitis, and colds. It is also useful for dry skin, eczema, psoriasis, impetigo, and sinusitis.

FOR THE MIND: benzoin eases insomnia, anxiety, panic attacks, and nightmares (especially in young children), and restores confidence.

BLENDS WELL WITH: frankincense, cedarwood, sandalwood, lavender, rosewood, geranium, orange, vetiver, lemon, melissa, cardamom, coriander, marjoram, neroli, bay, ginger, jasmine, myrrh, and rose.

Niaouli Melaleuca viridiflora

Niaouli is a relative of tea tree, and its traditional uses among Australian aboriginals included the clearing of respiratory and skin infections, coughs, colds, and headaches.

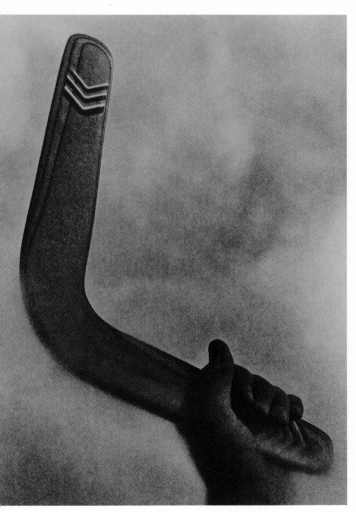

Niaouli is popular among Australian aboriginals, who use it to clear respiratory and skin infections. The essential oil is extracted from the leaves of the niaouli tree, which grows in Australia and the French West Indies.

DATA FILE

GROWN IN: Australia, Tasmania

IN A BLEND: 2 drops in 4 teaspoons/20 ml carrier oil (see pages 92–3)

FOR THE BODY: niaouli is a mild painkiller. It also helps to reduce blood pressure and stimulate the immune system. It is a very effective antiseptic and antiviral essential oil, and is useful in easing the symptoms associated with hemorrhoids, heart palpitations, varicose veins, diarrhea, flatulence, gastroenteritis, stomach ulcers, boils, eczema, dermatitis, cracked/dry skin, herpes simplex, insect bites and stings, psoriasis, asthma, bronchitis, catarrh, influenza, laryngitis, and sinusitis.

FOR THE MIND: niaouli is a stimulant and helps to combat apathy, boredom, discouragement, fear, forgetfulness, frustration, grief, irritability, and lethargy.

BLENDS WELL WITH: bay, benzoin, frankincense, pine, cedarwood, rosemary, lavender, marjoram, neroli, cypress, ylang ylang, clary sage, peppermint, ginger, yarrow, rose, geranium, lemon, grapefruit, vetiver, eucalyptus, tea tree, and thyme.

NIAOULI TREE

Bay laurel Pimenta acris

Bay's link with the mind dates back to its use as a visionary herb by the oracle at Delphi in Greece. Its leaves have been used to celebrate victory and achievement throughout Europe and the essential oil is a wonderful addition to a vaporizer to promote clear thinking and concentration.

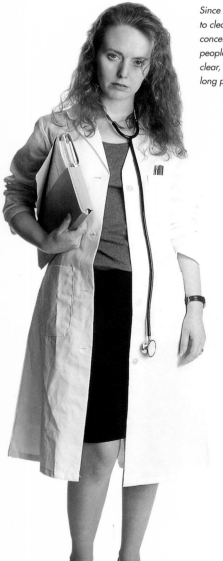

Since bay essential oil can help to clear the mind and improve concentration, it is very helpful for people in professions that require clear, focused concentration for long periods of time.

SAFETY NOTE
Do not use this essential oil on babies, toddlers, and older children.

DATA FILE

GROWN IN: South America, Antilles, Mexico, Venezuela, Barbados, Jamaica

IN A BLEND: 1 drop in 4 teaspoons/20 ml carrier oil (see pages 92–3)

FOR THE BODY: bay is an extremely effective antiseptic and antiviral essential oil. It is particularly useful for the respiratory system, easing the symptoms of coughs, colds, influenza, bronchitis, asthma, catarrh, and sinusitis.

FOR THE MIND: bay is useful for poor concentration, nervous exhaustion, and lack of energy or self-esteem. It also encourages lateral thinking and a creative approach to problem-solving.

BLENDS WELL WITH: benzoin, frankincense, cedarwood, rosewood, sandalwood, patchouli, vetiver, bergamot, grapefruit, orange, geranium, rose, niaouli, pine, tea tree, yarrow, marjoram, black pepper, and cardamom.

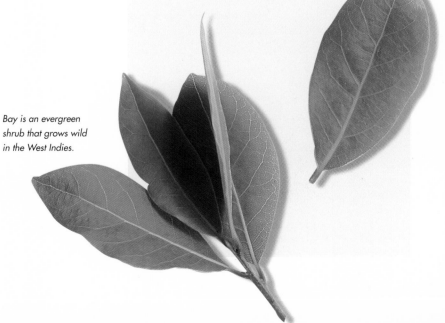

Bay is an evergreen shrub that grows wild in the West Indies.

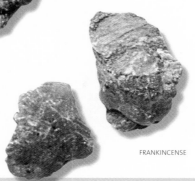

Frankincense
Boswellia carterii

FRANKINCENSE

F rankincense has been used in religious ceremonies for over 5,000 years. Frankincense's ability to instill calm and serenity is legendary. Its smooth, subtle, and resinous fragrance helps to prepare the mind for meditation and prayer, making it a popular ingredient in the incense used in many Jewish, Christian, and Hindu ceremonies today.

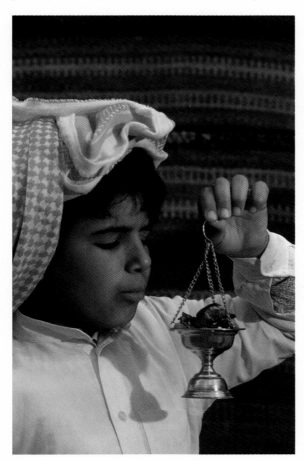

Frankincense has been used in many religious ceremonies around the world.

DATA FILE

GROWN IN: Somalia, North Africa, Ethiopia, Red Sea

IN A BLEND: 3 drops in 4 teaspoons/20 ml carrier oil (see pages 92–3)

FOR THE BODY: frankincense helps to repair wounds and is particularly useful to support the respiratory system and to ease muscular aches and pains. Use it for all forms of arthritis, colds, catarrh, laryngitis, dry or aging skin, heavy and painful periods, and endometriosis. It can also be used to support cancer treatment and to improve memory retention.

FOR THE MIND: use frankincense to restore confidence and for mental rejuvenation, comfort, to restore confidence and calm, and aging, fear, paranoia, nightmares, depression, and emotional exhaustion

BLENDS WELL WITH: rose, neroli, melissa, lemon, grapefruit, myrrh, cedarwood, benzoin, coriander, cardamom, rosemary, lemongrass, lavender, geranium, sandalwood, ylang ylang, yarrow, Roman camomile, and cypress.

SAFETY NOTE
unlikely to cause an
adverse reaction.

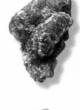

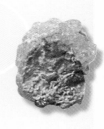

FRANKINCENSE

Abdominal massage

Abdominal massage is one of the most effective massages for reducing the pain associated with stress-related digestive problems such as bloating, constipation, diarrhea, and irritable bowel syndrome. It also eases painful periods. This massage is a wonderful way for expectant mothers to adjust to the changing shape of their bodies and to prevent stretchmarks.

Abdominal massage can help pregnant women to adjust to the changing shape of their bodies.

Since the abdomen is a very sensitive area, there are a couple of additional precautions involved in abdominal massage. Do not carry out deep (heavy) abdominal massage during pregnancy or during the first three days of menstruation. This will be uncomfortable, and in the latter case, may increase the flow of menstrual blood.

TIP

If the person you are massaging is experiencing a lot of abdominal pain, follow up your gentle abdominal massage with a hot water bottle or hot compress. The additional heat helps to encourage the essential oils to penetrate the skin more quickly. Remember, however, that abdominal pain can sometimes be an indication of something more serious. If you do not know the reason for the pain, always consult a doctor before turning to aromatherapy.

MASSAGING THE ABDOMEN

1 Apply the oil in smooth, circular strokes, moving in a clockwise direction from the stomach down the left side, across the hips, and up the right side of the body. Take in as much of the abdomen as you can. Repeat this smooth effleurage stroke (see page 49) between each of the other strokes.

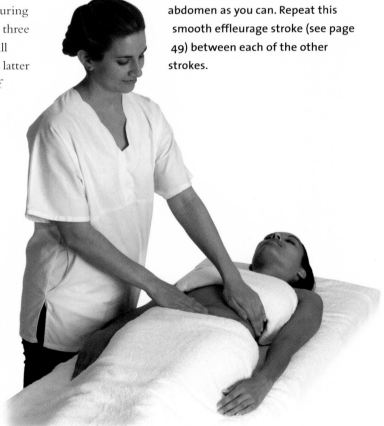

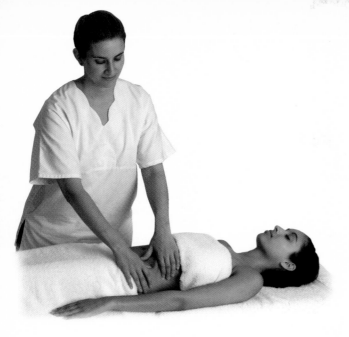

3 Placing your fingertips at the navel, glide your hands up the abdomen to the base of the sternum (breastbone), and follow the shape of the ribcage (along the bottom of the ribcage) as far around to the back as you can comfortably move your hands. Gently pull up, sliding your hands around the waist and back to the navel. Repeat three times. This is a lovely stretch to the lower back as well as massaging the stomach area.

2 Knead (see page 50) into the waist on both sides of the body. Really try to grasp the flesh and knead it out—this feels great and, with regular use, can enhance the shape of the waist.

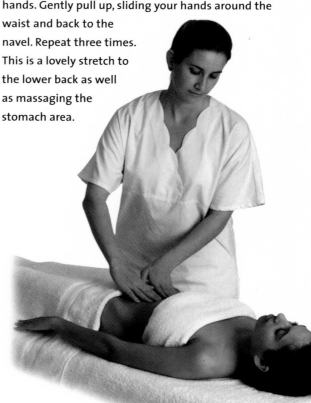

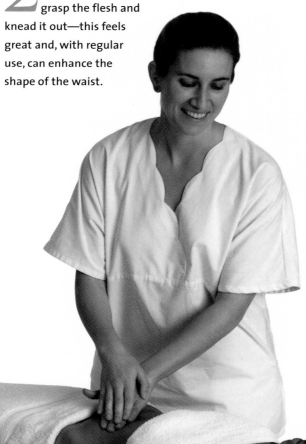

4 Use reinforced hands—place one hand over the other—so that your pressure will be a bit heavier. Move your hands in a rhythmic, wavelike circular pattern around the navel. This is very good for easing constipation. Repeat step 1 to finish.

Taking time to digest the problem: the **digestive** system

The delicate chemical balance within the digestive system is easily upset by a stressful lifestyle. Stress can slow down the digestion and absorption of food, but just as many problems arise if we skip meals or do not take time to sit down and eat properly.

Stress also leads many individuals to turn to sugary foods, caffeine, or alcohol for comfort, all of which have the potential to add more stress to the body's functioning or wreak havoc on their own. The increasing numbers of us suffering from irritable bowel syndrome, ulcers, food intolerances, and even diabetes suggests it is time we considered the quality of the food we are putting into our bodies, and how we prepare it. We also need to take time out to eat properly. The essential oils suggested here help to soothe abdominal discomfort and relieve the symptoms associated with a nervous digestive system. Turn to Roman camomile, geranium, yarrow, neroli, fennel, or peppermint in particular when you have "butterflies in your stomach" or you are faced with a problem you find hard to digest.

Too much sugar, caffeine, and alcohol can all upset the delicate balance of the digestive system.

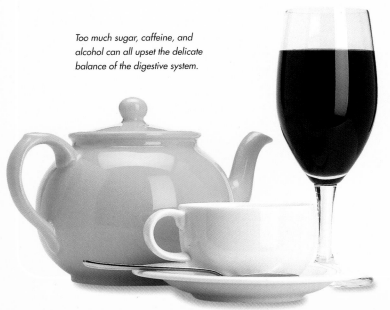

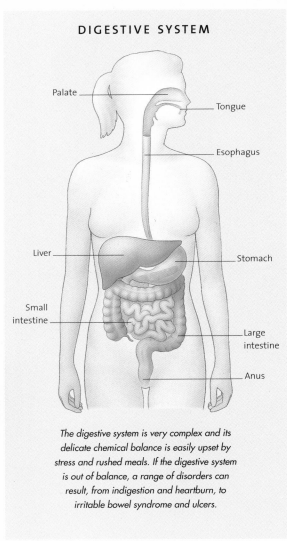

DIGESTIVE SYSTEM

Palate

Tongue

Esophagus

Liver

Stomach

Small intestine

Large intestine

Anus

The digestive system is very complex and its delicate chemical balance is easily upset by stress and rushed meals. If the digestive system is out of balance, a range of disorders can result, from indigestion and heartburn, to irritable bowel syndrome and ulcers.

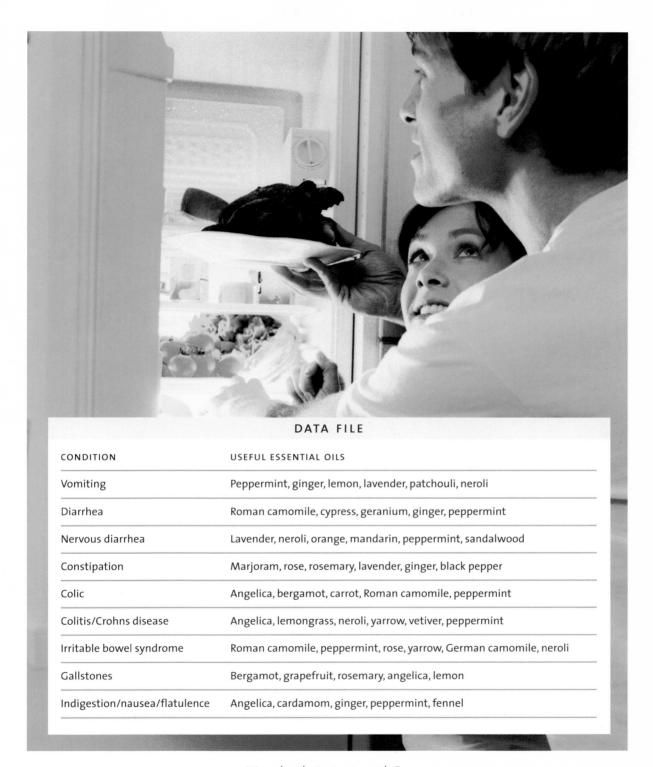

DATA FILE

CONDITION	USEFUL ESSENTIAL OILS
Vomiting	Peppermint, ginger, lemon, lavender, patchouli, neroli
Diarrhea	Roman camomile, cypress, geranium, ginger, peppermint
Nervous diarrhea	Lavender, neroli, orange, mandarin, peppermint, sandalwood
Constipation	Marjoram, rose, rosemary, lavender, ginger, black pepper
Colic	Angelica, bergamot, carrot, Roman camomile, peppermint
Colitis/Crohns disease	Angelica, lemongrass, neroli, yarrow, vetiver, peppermint
Irritable bowel syndrome	Roman camomile, peppermint, rose, yarrow, German camomile, neroli
Gallstones	Bergamot, grapefruit, rosemary, angelica, lemon
Indigestion/nausea/flatulence	Angelica, cardamom, ginger, peppermint, fennel

We need to take time to eat properly. Too many rushed meals or unhealthy foods will play havoc with the digestive system and can cause a variety of ailments.

Roman camomile
Anthemis nobilis

The essential oil is distilled from the dried flowers of the plant.

Roman camomile is one of the oldest known remedies. Fragments of it have been found in the excavations of Egyptian tombs and the herb was dedicated to the sun god, Ra. Later, it was also recommended by the Ancient Greek physician Hippocrates as a remedy for fevers. Roman camomile was an important plant in European herb gardens in the Middle Ages; it has been used as a strewing herb, as a tea to combat headaches and period pains, and as a cosmetic to lighten blonde hair.

Roman camomile was dedicated to the Egyptian sun god, Ra, and has been found in tomb excavations.

SAFETY NOTE unlikely to cause an adverse reaction.

DATA FILE

GROWN IN: England, Southern Europe, North America

IN A BLEND: 3 drops in 4 teaspoons/ 20 ml carrier oil (see pages 92–3)

FOR THE BODY: Roman camomile is an effective painkiller and anti-inflammatory agent. Use it for arthritis, colic, diarrhoea, flatulence, irritable bowel syndrome, indigestion, painful, irregular or heavy periods, premenstrual tension, discomfort associated with menopause, gastric reflux, nausea, vomiting, constipation, ulcers, eczema, boils, burns, stings, cracked nipples, poor appetite, anemia, intestinal parasites, epilepsy, headaches, migraines, neuralgia, and toothache.

FOR THE MIND: Roman camomile calms anger, insomnia, irritability, impatience, restlessness, resentment, nervous tension, shock, anxiety, and depression.

BLENDS WELL WITH: yarrow, marjoram, orange, benzoin, peppermint, geranium, rosemary, lemon, rose, neroli, fennel, clary sage, ginger, cedarwood, lavender, carrot seed, palmarosa, and bay.

Peppermint Mentha piperita

P eppermint's cool, clean flavor makes it one of the most popular ingredients in the food and cosmetic industry today. It has been used throughout the ages for everything from ceremonial incense to scenting bath water and bedlinens, and its fresh fragrance is an effective tonic for the mind, especially when faced with long-term anxiety or poor concentration.

SAFETY NOTE

can be slightly irritating to sensitive skin.

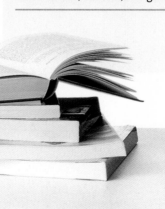

DATA FILE

GROWN IN: USA, Europe

IN A BLEND: 2 drops in 4 teaspoons/ 20 ml carrier oil (see pages 92–3)

FOR THE BODY: peppermint is useful for muscular aches and pains, arthritis, sprains, strains, acne, pruritis, poor circulation, varicose veins, colds, sinusitis, diarrhea, flatulence, gastritis, colitis, irritable bowel syndrome, indigestion, morning sickness, nausea, stomach cramps, vomiting, painful or swollen breasts, painful periods, lack of periods, headache, migraine, neuralgia, sciatica, toothache, fevers, and hangovers.

FOR THE MIND: peppermint is an effective stimulant. Use it for poor concentration and mental fatigue, and to improve memory retention, clear confusion, and improve decision making.

BLENDS WELL WITH: lemon, rosemary, lemongrass, yarrow, cedarwood, rosewood, Roman camomile, German camomile, cardamom, ginger, marjoram, carrot seed, basil, valerian, juniper, cypress, frankincense, tea tree, and geranium.

Peppermint essential oil helps to ease mental fatigue and improve powers of concentration, which is ideal for anyone studying for exams.

Hand and **arm** massage

This is a lovely massage to help ease conditions such as repetitive strain injury, and aching joints and muscles. It also has the added benefit of addressing a number of reflex points in the hands, thereby helping to reduce anxiety and stress elsewhere in the body.

1 Working from the wrist, apply oil in a smooth stroke that takes in the whole of the arm and shoulder. Return to the wrist and repeat up to three times.

STEP 1

STEP 3

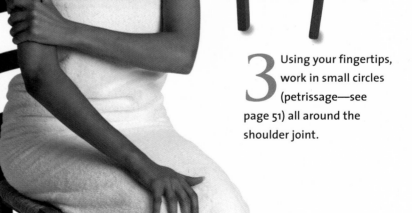

2 Knead the whole of the arm (see page 50), working first over the forearm before moving on to the upper arm. Spend most of the time on the upper arm—this movement is very good for helping to tone the upper arm muscles.

STEP 2

3 Using your fingertips, work in small circles (petrissage—see page 51) all around the shoulder joint.

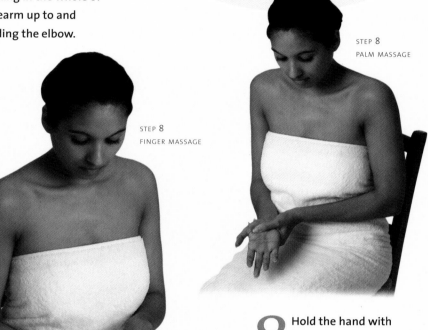

4 Using the same movement, work in small circles from the wrist bones all along the forearm. This is particularly good if someone suffers from poor circulation or repetitive strain injury. Be as slow and detailed over this area as you can be, taking in the whole of the forearm up to and including the elbow.

STEP 4

TIP
Carrier oils are excellent for improving the health and strength of the fingernails—if your nails break easily or seem to take forever to grow, massage your hands regularly with oil. You will see significant improvements in a matter of weeks. See pages 92–3 for a selection of carrier oils.

STEP 8
PALM MASSAGE

STEP 8
FINGER MASSAGE

5 Using the whole of the side of your thumb, gently squeeze it along the side of the forearm. This helps to encourage any swelling in this area to return to the circulation system.

6 Lift and support the elbow, then repeat step 6 for the upper arm.

7 Repeat step 1, this time taking in the whole of the hand as well as the arm and shoulder. Repeat up to three times.

8 Hold the hand with the palm facing upward. Use your thumbs to work in small, deep circles over the entire palm. Pay particular attention to the center of the palm, the heel of the hand, and also the base of the thumb.
Hold the hand with the palm facing downward, and use your fingertips to knead each finger in turn
Repeat step 1 to finish.

Getting rid of that pain in the neck:
muscular aches and pains

When combined with massage, aromatherapy is exceptionally good at easing aching muscles. A large majority of people experiencing stress will complain of muscular aches and pains, particularly in their necks, shoulders, back, and upper arms. Whether we are aware of it or not, we instinctively hunch or curl up when we are under stress, crouching over computer screens, telephones, or household chores for many hours of the day. Good posture, a change in the way your work station is set up, massage, or the Alexander technique can all combine to reduce the aches and pains associated with stress. The essential oils suggested here all help to reduce pain and relax over-contracted muscles. Regular aromatherapy massage and warm baths can help to keep your muscles in excellent condition.

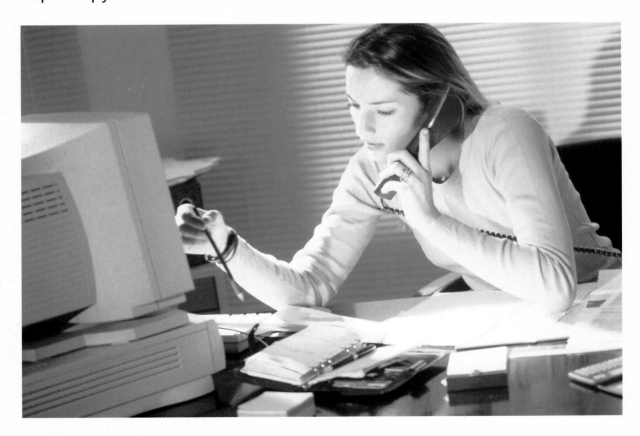

DATA FILE

CONDITION	USEFUL ESSENTIAL OILS
Muscular aches and pains	Basil, black pepper, carrot seed, cinnamon, clove, eucalyptus, frankincense, ginger, lemongrass, marjoram, peppermint, rosemary, vetiver
Muscular spasms	Basil, bay, carrot seed, cinnamon, clove, German camomile, lavender, marjoram, valerian, vetiver
Sprains (of muscles or tendons) strains (of ligaments)	Eucalyptus, German camomile, ginger, peppermint, rosemary, yarrow, Roman camomile
Arthritis	Basil, black pepper, carrot seed, cypress, eucalyptus, German camomile, grapefruit, ginger, lavender, lemongrass, lemon, melissa
Repetitive strain injury	Basil, black pepper, carrot seed, clove, cinnamon, German camomile, ginger, peppermint, Roman camomile
Tension headaches and migraines	Basil, carrot seed, frankincense, grapefruit, lavender, lemon, marjoram, melissa, Roman camomile, yarrow, ylang ylang`

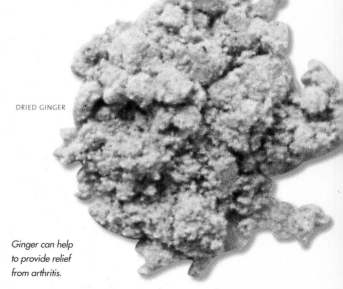

Essential oils such as eucalyptus, ginger, peppermint, and rosemary can ease the pain of sports injuries, including sprains and strained ligaments.

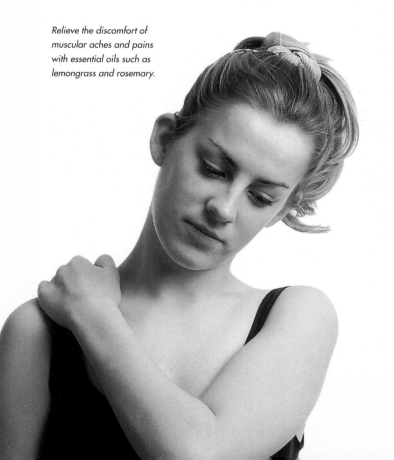

Relieve the discomfort of muscular aches and pains with essential oils such as lemongrass and rosemary.

DRIED GINGER

Ginger can help to provide relief from arthritis.

In some cultures, yarrow is used to help determine feelings of love and loyalty.

Yarrow Achillea millefolium

This quiet, pretty inhabitant of many European cottage gardens has led an interesting life. Its stalks were once used to practice a form of divination in China known as *I Ching*. Yarrow has been widely used through history to staunch wounds and, in some cultures, as a method of determining feelings of love, loyalty, and fidelity.

Yarrow is used for medicine and divination in some cultures.

Yarrow is a common plant and grows in the wild.

DATA FILE

GROWN IN: Germany, Hungary, Yugoslavia

IN A BLEND: 2 drops in 4 teaspoons/20 ml carrier oil (see pages 92–3)

FOR THE BODY: yarrow is an extremely effective painkiller, antispasmodic, and anti-inflammatory oil. It is particularly useful in the treatment of rheumatoid arthritis, dermatitis, eczema, pruritis, skin inflammations, cirrhosis, colitis, hemorrhoids, inflammations of the stomach, kidney, bladder, and colon, peptic ulcers, oral and vaginal thrush, incontinence, prostatitis, epilepsy, allergies, chronic fatigue, and muscular aches and pains.

FOR THE MIND: yarrow is an effective sedative. Use it to combat insomnia, anger, irritability, anxiety, resentment, sexual overexcitement, tearfulness, and frustration, and to aid recovery from alcohol addiction.

BLENDS WELL WITH: rose, rosemary, rosewood, Roman camomile, German camomile, lavender, geranium, lemon, grapefruit, peppermint, cypress, sandalwood, cedarwood, melissa, fennel, palmarosa, ylang ylang, frankincense, lemongrass, ginger, basil, and marjoram.

SAFETY NOTE
photosensitive— may cause skin rash

Vetiver Vetiveria zizanoides

Vetiver is used extensively in the Far East to create fans, curtains, and mats. Its woody fragrance helps to repel insects as well as relieving headaches and fever. It is also a popular ingredient in men's colognes. Vetiver is, in fact, a wild grass and the essential oil is distilled from its roots. It has a distinctive sweet aroma.

Vetiver is an aphrodisiac and helps to restore lost sex drive. It also helps women to conceive and prepares the body for labor.

DATA FILE

GROWN IN: Haiti, Réunion, Java, China

IN A BLEND: 2 drops in 4 teaspoons/20 ml of carrier oil

FOR THE BODY: vetiver is closely linked with the liver and the muscular and reproductive systems. It is effective at easing muscular spasms, lymphatic congestion, constipation, and colitis, and aiding liver regeneration following alcohol addiction. It also stimulates reproductive function in women trying to conceive; during the last three months of pregnancy, it prepares the body for labor.

FOR THE MIND: vetiver is a euphoric and sedating essential oil. It is also an effective aphrodisiac and helps ease symptoms associated with lack of sexual interest, insecurity, lack of confidence or warmth, defeatism, inability to relax, insomnia, sluggishness, and recovery from addiction.

BLENDS WELL WITH: frankincense, rose, geranium, sandalwood, palmarosa, orange, lavender, lemongrass, bergamot, grapefruit, Roman camomile, ginger, peppermint, clary sage, fennel, juniper, melissa, and neroli.

VETIVER

SAFETY NOTE unlikely to cause an adverse reaction.

Leg and **foot** massage

You can adapt this treatment to massage your own legs. This is a very effective way of stimulating circulation to the legs and feet, improving skin and muscle tone, reducing the appearance of cellulite, and reducing swelling and lymphatic congestion.

MASSAGING THE LEGS AND FEET

1 Expose the back of the leg and apply oil, using smooth long effleurage strokes (see page 49) along the length of the leg, up to the point at which the towel stops, then bring both hands lightly down the outside of the leg. Repeat this several times, to warm up the leg.

2 Knead the whole of the thigh area (see page 50), concentrating on working on the outside of the leg in particular. Really work into the muscles so that they warm up thoroughly (the skin may sometimes redden slightly as you do this).

3 Use your knuckles to work deeper into the muscles. Remember to use only the first knuckle of your fingers, putting your weight onto your hands and then rotating your hands from the wrists.

4 Knead the calf muscles in the same way as for step 2. Really work into the muscles.

5 Use your fingertips to work in small circles around the back of the ankle and to either side of the Achilles tendon (at the back of the calf).

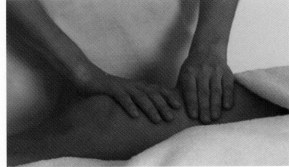

STEP 1

STEP 2

STEP 6

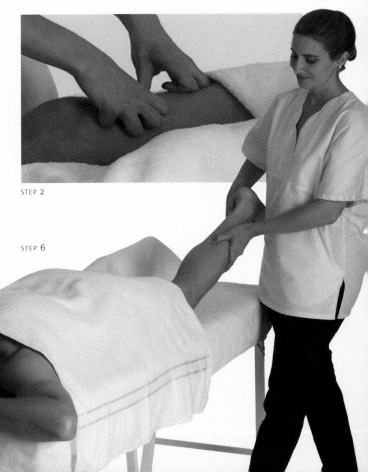

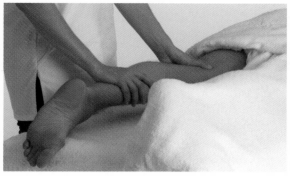

STEP 7

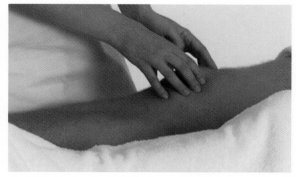

STEP 12

6 Bend the knee. Use the side of your thumb to "drain" the lower leg from the ankle to the back of the knee. This is a form of lymphatic drainage that eases congestion and swelling in the legs.

7 Lower the knee and then repeat the drainage movement to the back of the thigh. If you press hard enough, you will sometimes find small fatty deposits in the mid thigh area—it will feel as if you are "popping" bubble wrap as you go over the area.

8 Repeat effleurage as for Step 1, cover the leg, then repeat steps 1–7 for the other leg.

9 Turn the person over, expose the front of the leg, and apply oil using effleurage as for step 1. Lift your hands slightly as you go over the knee area. This can sometimes be painful if you press too hard.

10 Knead the whole of the thigh area, concentrating on the outer thigh. Knuckle the whole of the thigh area.

11 Use the heel of your hand to "drain" the outer area of the thigh from the knee up to the hip (the edge of the towel).

12 Work with the fingers in small circles around the knee, then bring your hands smoothly down the front of the leg to the ankle. Repeat these small circles around the ankle.

13 Squeeze the foot between your hands, pushing your hands down the foot from the toes to the heel.

14 Run your fingers in strips down the front of the foot, slotting your fingers in between the bones of the foot.

15 Run your fingers in strips under the foot, from the base of each toe to the ankle.

16 Make a light fist. Press it just under the ball of the foot. Push down and move your fist from the ball of the foot to the heel.

17 Repeat the long effleurage movements carried out in step 9 over the whole leg. Repeat steps 9–17 for the other leg.

STEP 14

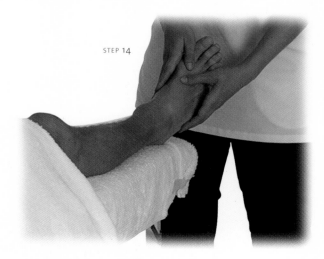

Time to put your feet up:
stress-related **circulation** disorders

Stress can have pronounced effects on the circulation of blood and lymph around the body. If you are on your feet, rushing around most of the day, not only will you find that your feet hurt, but sometimes this is accompanied by swelling in your legs and ankles or the development of varicose veins. Elsewhere, you might notice that cellulite deposits seem to be increasing on your legs. Alternatively, you might find that you develop poor circulation, with your hands and/or feet feeling constantly cold.

S tress can also lead to changes in blood pressure: usually blood pressure will go up when you are under stress. Some of the contributing factors to raised blood pressure include alcohol, caffeine, and nicotine intake, weight gain (through additional food intake and also through pregnancy), taking the contraceptive pill, aging, diet, and most importantly, a lifestyle high in stress.

As well as turning to aromatherapy, there are a number of simple things you can do to reduce the effects of stress on your circulation system. Take time out to put your feet up

After a busy day, try to put your feet up. If necessary, spray your legs and feet with alternating hot and cold water to soothe and revive them.

after a busy day—this will help to reduce swelling in your legs and ankles. You can reduce the appearance of varicose veins, or prominent veins in your legs that look like they might become varicose, by spraying them with alternating hot and cold water at the end of your daily shower. Simply take the shower attachment off the wall and hold it close to the backs of your legs, or wherever the varicose veins have appeared. Spray cold water against them for 30 seconds, then warm water for 30 seconds, and repeat for a couple of minutes. This helps to tone the muscles in the walls of the blood vessels, and will improve your circulation generally.

A busy, stressful lifestyle can have negative effects on your circulation and can lead to complaints ranging from varicose veins to heart palpitations.

DATA FILE

CONDITION	USEFUL ESSENTIAL OILS
Hypertension— high blood pressure	Carrot seed, geranium, jasmine, lavender, spikenard, valerian, and ylang ylang
Hypotension — low blood pressure	Lemongrass, peppermint, and rosemary
Heart palpitations	Frankincense, spikenard, and ylang ylang
Reynaud's Syndrome, poor circulation	Black pepper, cypress, geranium, lavender, lemongrass, and rosemary
Cellulite	Angelica, bergamot, cypress, grapefruit, lemon, lemongrass, juniper and rosemary
Varicose veins, hemorrhoids, thread veins, broken veins	Black pepper, cypress, lemon, lavender, neroli, niaouli, myrrh, pine, and yarrow

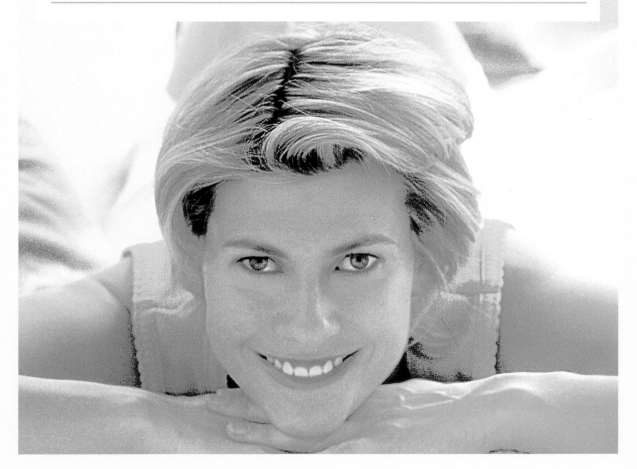

Spikenard
Nardostachys jatamansi

Spikenard's warm earthy fragrance and its ability to soothe anxiety have made it a key ingredient in religious ceremonies and it has been used to anoint both secular and religious leaders for generations. There are frequent references to it as "nard" in the Bible, which include Mary Magdalene anointing Jesus with it before the Last Supper.

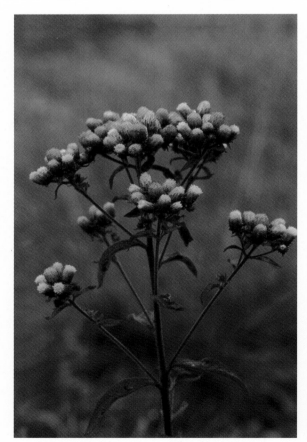

Spikenard has been an important ingredient in religious rituals around the world.

The essential oil is very soothing and helps to stabilize mood swings. It also eases insomnia.

DATA FILE

GROWN IN: India, Nepal

IN A BLEND: 2 drops in 4 teaspoons/20 ml of carrier oil (see pages 92–3)

FOR THE BODY: spikenard is a strong antispasmodic and anticonvulsive oil, and is useful for for heart problems such as palpitations, irregular heart beats, and high blood pressure. It also provides useful support in the treatment of epilepsy. It is also useful for nausea, constipation, premenstrual tension, lack of periods, and also painful periods.

FOR THE MIND: spikenard is very effective for insomnia, mood swings, irritability, panic attacks, and nervous exhaustion.

BLENDS WELL WITH: rose, neroli, palmarosa, vetiver, sandalwood, ylang ylang, nutmeg, ginger, geranium, and damiana.

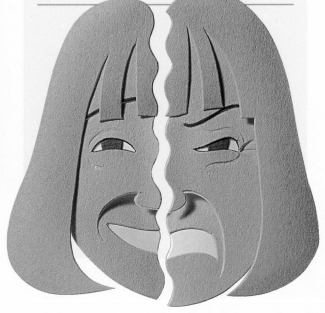

Black pepper

Piper nigrum

Black pepper stimulates the immune system. Combine it with tea tree and lemon to aid recovery from colds and flu.

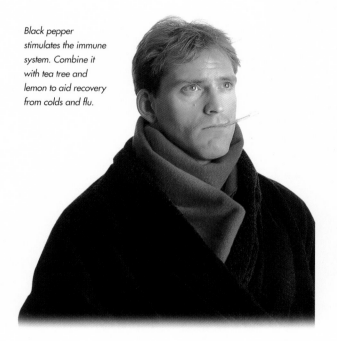

Black pepper vines grow in the Far East. The fruit's medicinal value is prized by homeopaths and Ayurvedic practitioners too.

B lack pepper was once a valuable commodity in the ancient spice trade, and has been used throughout history to support people engaged in lengthy travel or feats of endurance because it was thought to increase stamina. Its hot, spicy aroma warms the heart and stimulates the immune system. Try it with lemon and tea tree essential oils to get you on your feet again after a cold.

SAFETY NOTE

unlikely to cause an adverse reaction. Black pepper raises blood pressure.

DATA FILE

GROWN IN: Indonesia, China, India, Madagascar

IN A BLEND: 3 drops in 4 teaspoons/20 ml carrier oil (see pages 92–3)

FOR THE BODY: black pepper is a very effective painkiller, antispasmodic, and antiviral essential oil. Black pepper is also useful for people with low blood pressure, and is helpful for muscular aches and pains, arthritis, cold sores, poor circulation, colds, constipation, diarrhea, flatulence, loss of appetite, nausea, sluggish digestion, postviral fatigue, lack of appetite, edema (swelling), influenza, and tonsillitis.

FOR THE MIND: black pepper is a stimulant and aphrodisiac. Use it to help people who are feeling apathetic, sluggish, lacking in energy, or recovering from eating disorders, or suffering from depression or chronic anxiety.

BLENDS WELL WITH: neroli, rosemary, rose, bergamot, tea tree, lavender, orange, cardamom, ginger, lemongrass, marjoram, peppermint, lemon, grapefruit, frankincense, geranium, sandalwood, cedarwood, Roman camomile, and yarrow.

Juniper Juniperus communis

The clean, astringent fragrance of juniper has been used throughout history as a ceremonial incense, to prevent infection, and to keep away vermin. Juniper is one of the key ingredients in the manufacture of gin, and is also a popular food flavoring.

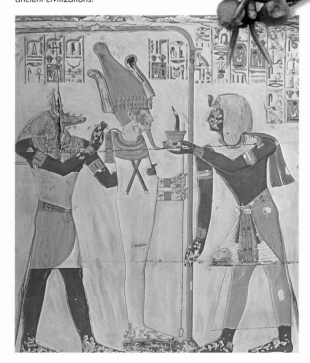

The juniper bush grows in Europe and the USA.

Juniper was prized as a purifying, stimulating ceremonial incense by ancient civilizations.

DATA FILE

GROWN IN: Italy, Yugoslavia, USA

IN A BLEND: 3 drops in 4 teaspoons/20 ml carrier oil (see pages 92–3)

FOR THE BODY: juniper is an unparalleled diuretic, antiseptic, and general tonic, and clears toxins throughout the body. Use it for arteriosclerosis, gout, rheumatoid arthritis, oily skin, skin disorders, edema (swelling), poor circulation, coughs, colds, painful and absent periods, cystitis, prostatitis, and urinary stones.

FOR THE MIND: juniper clears and stimulates the mind, prevents worry and unpleasant memories, and renews optimism and zest for life. Use it when you need to clear the atmosphere in a room or if you are expecting visitors who leave you feeling exhausted.

BLENDS WELL WITH: frankincense, myrrh, cypress, lemon, grapefruit, orange, lavender, yarrow, sandalwood, geranium, rose, vetiver, angelica, black pepper, tea tree, and jasmine.

SAFETY NOTE
avoid juniper if suffering from a kidney infection or disease or when taking diuretics.

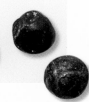

JUNIPER BERRIES

Cypress Cupressus sempervirens

A long association with death and grieving has led cypress trees to be planted in graveyards all over Europe. Their mildly astringent aroma helps to comfort the bereaved, encouraging them to let go of grief and anger and let optimism and peace of mind return.

Cypress trees are traditionally planted in European cemeteries.

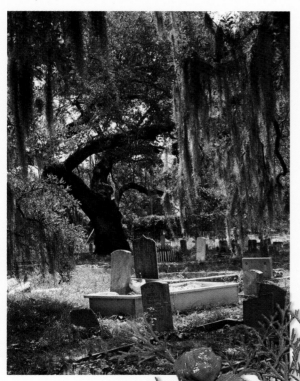

Add a few drops of cypress essential oil to the water reservoir of an oil burner in a room to soothe the nervous system and ease tension.

DATA FILE

GROWN IN: France, Spain, Morocco

IN A BLEND: 3 drops in 4 teaspoons/20 ml carrier oil (see pages 92–3)

FOR THE BODY: cypress' astringent properties and close link with the cardiovascular system make it extremely useful for reducing the effects of broken, red, and thread veins, oily skin, acne, boils, cysts, polyps, fibroids, cellulite, joint pain, hemorrhoids and varicose veins. It is also very useful in treating respiratory conditions such as asthma, coughs, colds, emphysema, influenza and watery colds, as well as heavy and painful periods, cystitis, fluid retention, incontinence, loose stools, colitis and excessive perspiration.

FOR THE MIND: cypress provides very effective support for restlessness, depression, nervous exhaustion, overtalkativeness, anxiety, frustration, bereavement, and self-doubt.

BLENDS WELL WITH: juniper, geranium, myrrh, frankincense, marjoram, neroli, basil, clove, nutmeg, cedarwood, sandalwood, rosemary, tea tree, lavender, orange, grapefruit, yarrow, benzoin, pine, and niaouli.

SAFETY NOTE
unlikely to cause an adverse reaction.

CYPRESS

SWEET ALMOND OIL

SWEET ALMONDS

Carrier oils

Aromatherapists use carrier oils literally to "carry" the essential oil, spreading them lightly over the body of the person receiving treatment. Essential oils dissolve most effectively in vegetable oils, and while any vegetable oil could be used as a carrier oil, each one has particular properties that can enhance the treatment, especially when treating skin conditions.

AVOCADO

This table gives you more detail about some of the most popular carrier oils. It is certainly worth investing in more than one variety because you can blend the carrier oils themselves as well. For a more enriching massage oil, try adding 1 teaspoon/5 ml of avocado or jojoba oil to 3 teaspoons/15 ml of a lighter oil such as grapeseed or sweet almond. For extremely luxurious facial blends, why not use avocado or jojoba as carrier oils on their own?

AVOCADO OIL

WHEAT GERM OIL

WHEAT GERM

TIP

Carrier oils can sometimes stain towels and clothes. For effective cleaning, use a biological liquid detergent in your washing machine and clean the towels and clothing you use for massage at the hottest possible setting (usually 194°f/90°c). Products used for cleaning babies' napkins are also an effective option.

MARIGOLD PETALS

CALENDULA OIL (FROM MARIGOLD PETALS)

DATA FILE

CARRIER OIL	PROPERTIES	USES
Avocado (*Persea americana*)	Can penetrate the upper layer of skin and is extremely therapeutic for dry and aging skin. Blend it with other carrier oils, such as grapeseed to enrich your blend.	Excellent moisturizer for dry or dehydrated skin and fine, aging skin, or for eczema and psoriasis. Choose an unrefined oil if possible—look for its dark green color.
Calendula (*Calendula officinalis*)	Known for its wound-healing properties, calendula is a very light oil and, with dry skin, might be best used in combination with something like jojoba to enrich it.	Fades stretchmarks, reduces scar tissue and scarring from acne, and heals rashes and chapped or cracked skin.
Grapeseed (*Vitis vinifera*)	Light, non-greasy, absorbs into skin quickly, and unlikely to stain clothes.	A good all-purpose massage oil and very cost-effective. Use instead of sweet almond oil if you suffer from nut allergies.
Jojoba (*Simmondsia chinensis*)	Dissolves sebum and unclogs pores. Jojoba is a liquid wax and keeps well. Its chemical structure resembles sebum and sebum can dissolve in it, making it effective against acne. It can also be used for dry skin conditions such as eczema and dandruff. It also has slight anti-inflammatory properties.	Reduces fine lines, maintains health of aging skin, and clears acne. Jojoba can also help to preserve the blend, increasing its shelf-life.
Macadamia nut (*Macadamia integrifolia*)	Very nourishing and easily absorbed, this oil leaves skin feeling silky after treatment. Good for use in the bath, but expensive.	Absolutely excellent massage oil, which is particularly appropriate for dry, dehydrated or cracked skin.
Wheat germ (*Triticum vulgare*)	Very high in vitamin E; an excellent oil for treating eczema, red veins, and fine lines.	Useful on dry, aging skins and for eczema and psoriasis. It helps extend the shelf life of other blends (add up to 1 teaspoon/5 ml) to your main carrier oil). Do not use this carrier oil on people with wheat allergies.
Sunflower (*Helianthus annus*)	This oil is absorbed well. It is diuretic and high in unsaturated fatty acids, so it is good for leg ulcers, arteriosclerosis, skin diseases, and bruises. It contains inulin, which is used to treat asthma.	Sunflower is a good, cost-effective massage oil. It has a high vitamin E content, making it very useful for people with aging, dry, or dehydrated skin.
Sweet almond (*Prunus amygdalis*)	This oil has some vitamin E, so it keeps well and protects and nourishes the skin.	This is a good all-purpose massage oil and is good for dry, delicate, or sensitive skin.

Useful addresses

For a list of qualified aromatherapists in your area, see below:

American Alliance of Aromatherapy
P.O. Box 750428
Petaluma
CA 94975-0428

American Aromatherapy Association
P.O. Box 3679
South Pasadena
CA 91031

National Association for Holistic Aromatherapy
4509 Interlake Ave N 233
Seattle
WA 981093-2680
www.naha.org

Real Essences Aromatherapy
2122b MacDonald Street
Vancouver
British Columbia
V6K 3Y4
Canada

Nature Trading Limited
Box 263
1857 West 4th Avenue
B.C.V63 1M4
Canada

FOR AROMATHERAPY TRAINING:

International Therapies Examinations Council
ITEC courses in Massage and Aromatherapy are run at many colleges in Britain, Europe, South Africa, the Far East, Australia and New Zealand. For details of courses available near you, visit the ITEC website—
www.itecworld.co.uk

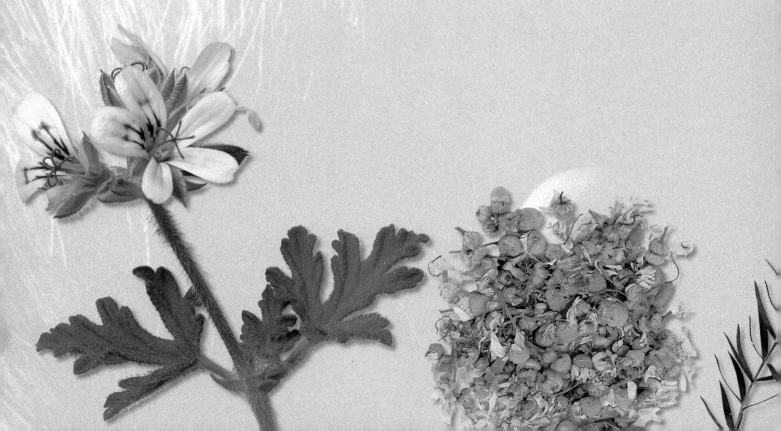